Essential Safety & Health at Work in Healthcare

Róisín Quínn

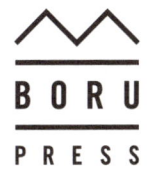

BORU PRESS

Boru Press Ltd.
The Farmyard
Birdhill
Co. Tipperary
www.borupress.ie

© Róisín Quínn 2020

ISBN 978 19160 1996 6

Design by Sarah McCoy
Print origination by Carole Lynch
Illustrations by Andriy Yankovskyy and Derry Dillon (Pg. 142)
Printed by GraphyCems Ltd, Spain

The paper used in this book is made from wood pulp of managed forests. For every tree felled, at least one tree is planted, thereby renewing natural resources.

All rights reserved. No part of this publication may be copied, reproduced or transmitted in any form or by any means without written permission of the publishers or else under the terms of any licence permitting limited copyright issued by the Irish Copyright Licensing Agency.

A CIP catalogue record for this book is available from the British Library.

For permission to reproduce photographs and artworks, the author and publisher gratefully acknowledge the following:

Homecare Medical Supplies 51, 127. Health and Safety Authority 3, 4, 25, 134, 135, 172. iStock 60, 61, 87, 88, 89, 100, 101, 104, 105, 126, 127, 130, 132, 139, 145. Róisín Quínn 19. Shutterstock 128.

The author and publisher have made every effort to trace all copyright holders, but if any has been inadvertently overlooked we would be pleased to make the necessary arrangement at the first opportunity.

CONTENTS

1 Health and Safety Legislation — 1

Health and Safety Legislation — 2
Healthcare Regulators — 3
Duties of Employers and Employees — 5
The Safety Statement — 9

2 A Safe and Healthy Work Environment — 13

Healthcare Injury Statistics in Ireland — 14
Maintaining a Safe and Healthy Work Environment — 15
Accidents and Incidents — 20
Recording and Reporting — 23

3 Risk Assessment — 29

What is a Risk Assessment? — 29
Why Perform a Risk Assessment? — 31
Performing a Risk Assessment — 33
Lone Workers — 44
Night Work and Shift Work — 45
Younger Workers — 46

4 Hazards in the Workplace — 49

Physical Hazards — 50
Chemical Hazards — 52
Psychosocial Hazards — 53
Biological Hazards — 58

Sharps	62
Safety Data Sheet (SDS)	65

5 Occupational Health Risks   68

Noise	68
Fumes and Dust	69
Protecting the Skin	71
Manual Handling	74
Mechanical Equipment	77
Electrical Equipment	78

6 Fire Prevention   80

Employer and Employee Responsibilities in Fire Prevention	81
The Fire Triangle	82
Ignition Sources	83
How Fire Spreads	84
Extinguishing a Fire	85
Fire-fighting Equipment	86
Fire Evacuation Procedures	89

7 Infection Prevention and Control   98

Microbiology	98
Pathogens	99
Types of Micro-Organism	99
Growth and Development of Micro-organisms	102
Spread of Micro-organisms	103
Infections	106
Healthcare-Associated Infections (HCAIs)	108
Preventive Measures and Emergency Procedures for Suspected Contamination	115
Healthcare Linen	119

8 Safety Equipment — 122
Personal Protective Equipment (PPE) — 122
First Aid Kit — 129
Automated External Defibrillator (AED) — 132
Safety Signs — 132

9 Communication and Training — 136
Communication — 136
Training — 147

10 Personal Health in the Workplace — 150
Safe and Healthy Working Practices — 150
A Safety Culture — 151
Safe Working Environments — 153
Risk Factors in Relation to Health — 156
Promoting Safety and Health in the Workplace — 162

Glossary of Health and Safety Terms — 166

Appendices — 167
1. Sample Accident/Incident Report Form — 167
2. Sample of Completed Risk Assessment: Slips, Trips and Falls — 169
3. Hazard Signs — 170

References and Further Reading — 171

Index — 180

List of Legislation and Regulations — 185

Dedication

This book is dedicated to my Grandad, Matty Quinn

"Don't dream your life, live your dreams" – Bob Bitchin

Acknowledgements:

I would like to thank Marion O'Brien at Boru Press for her support and guidance throughout the process of writing this book.

I would like to express my sincere thanks to my parents Christina and Matthew and my siblings Áine, Searlait and Matthew for their constant encouragement throughout my career.

To Christopher, who planted the seed to pursue my passion for teaching in the first place. Thank you for your patience and guidance and always believing in me and for inspiring me to be the best I can be.

I would like to extend a special thank you to my colleagues in VTOS, Limerick Clare ETB for their encouragement and guidance.

For the purpose of consistency the term 'client' is used in this book to refer to the person receiving care. In nursing homes they are usually referred to as 'residents', in homecare they may be referred to as 'clients', in hospitals they are referred to as 'patients' and in intellectual disability settings they are often referred to as 'service users'.

chapter 1
HEALTH AND SAFETY LEGISLATION

IN THIS CHAPTER YOU WILL LEARN ABOUT:

- The role of the Health and Safety Authority
- The safety statement
- The duties of employers and employees as specified in current safety, health and welfare at work legislation

Workplace health and safety has always been important, but it has become increasingly so in recent times. In the healthcare sector, the rising numbers of employees (294,300 workers in the health and social work sector in the first quarter of 2019) and service users underlines the importance of effective health and safety management in preventing and reducing healthcare workers' exposure to work hazards.

(CSO 2019)

The health and social work sector reports approximately 1,400 injuries each year to the Health and Safety Authority (HSA), accounting for nearly 20 per cent of all workplace injuries reported annually.

There are three main accident triggers in the healthcare sector:

1. Manual handling (client handling and handling of inanimate loads)

2. Slips, trips and falls (on the level)
3. Work-related shock, fright and violence.

(HSA 2015)

Clearly, healthcare is an area where safety and health protocols and procedures must be central to management plans and to all day-to-day activities.

> The **Safety, Health and Welfare at Work Act 2005** is the principal legislation providing for the health and safety of people in the workplace in Ireland.

Health and Safety Legislation

The principal legislation providing for the health and safety of people in the workplace is the **Safety, Health and Welfare at Work Act 2005**. This Act applies to all employers, employees (including fixed-term and temporary employees) and self-employed people in their workplaces. It sets out the rights and responsibilities of both employers and employees and provides for substantial fines and penalties for breaches of the health and safety legislation.

Health and safety legislation, policies and procedures are in place for the protection of both staff and service users. The **Safety, Health and Welfare at Work Act 2005** sets out the main provisions for organisations to secure and improve the safety, health and welfare of people at work. These include:

+ The management and organisation of the systems of work necessary to achieve a safe working environment

+ The requirements for the control of safety, health and welfare at work

- The identification of responsibilities and roles of employers and employees.

(HSE website)

If policies, procedures and legislation are not followed by the employer and the employees, unfavourable consequences will be realised, ranging from serious injury or death and legal proceedings in a court of law. The **Safety, Health and Welfare at Work Act 2005** and its amendments can be downloaded from the Irish Statute Book website, www.irishstatutebook.ie (search for Safety, Health and Welfare at Work Act 2005).

Healthcare Regulators

The Health and Safety Authority

The Health and Safety Authority (HSA) was established in 1989 under the Safety, Health and Welfare at Work Act 1989 (now replaced by the 2005 Act) and reports to the Minister of State under delegated authority from the Minister for Business, Enterprise and Innovation.

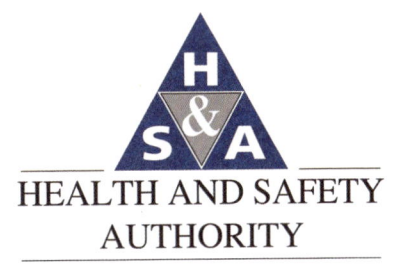

According to the HSA's Strategic Statement 2019-2021, Its vision is for healthy, safe and productive lives and enterprises in Ireland. Its mission is to work to ensure that duty holders meet their legal obligations in relation to workplace health and safety, market surveillance and chemicals. It also works to motivate and inform through a combination of promotion, information, education, inspection and enforcement activities.

Set out in over 200 Acts, regulations and international conventions, the legislative role of the HSA is to:

- Protect workers from occupational injury and illness
- Protect human health and the environment
- Enhance competitiveness and innovation
- Ensure the free movement of chemicals on the internal market
- Protect workers and the public from unsafe articles and products
- Accredit organisations to international standards for technical competence in testing, calibration, inspection, verification and certification.

The HSA has 5 strategic priorities:

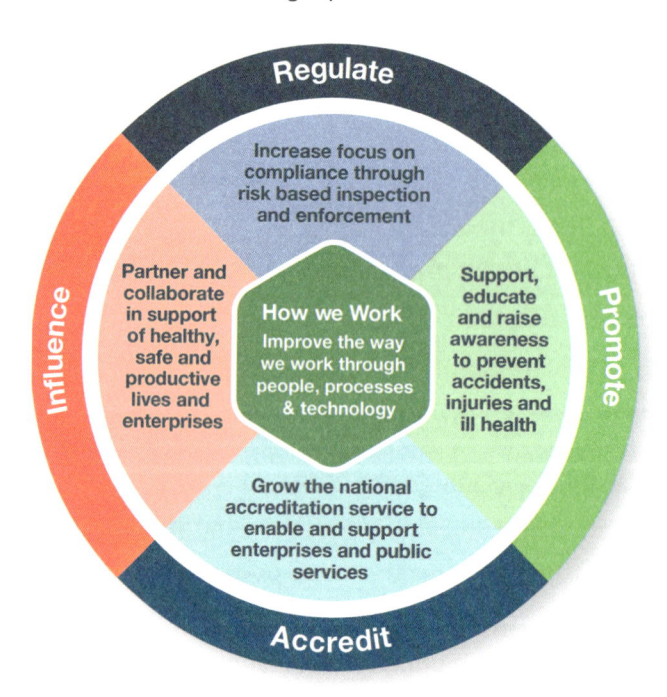

(HSA, 2019)

Other Healthcare Regulators

Other statutory bodies that regulate healthcare and their areas of responsibility are outlined below.

Regulators of services:

- Health and Information Quality Authority (HIQA) – *www.hiqa.ie*
- Mental Health Commission (MHC) – *www.mhcirl.ie*

Regulators of professionals:

- Nursing and Midwifery Board of Ireland (NMBI) – *www.nmbi.ie*
- Dental Council of Ireland – *www.dentalcouncil.ie*
- Health and Social Care Professionals Council (CORU) – *www.coru.ie*
- Medical Council of Ireland – *www.medicalcouncil.ie*
- Optical Registration Board – *www.coru.ie*
- Pharmaceutical Society of Ireland (PSI) – *www.thepsi.ie*
- Pre-Hospital Emergency Care Council (PHECC) – *www.phecit.ie*

Regulators of products:

- Food Safety Authority of Ireland (FSAI) – *www.fsai.ie*
- Health Products Regulatory Authority (HPRA) – *www.hpra.ie*
- Radiological Protection Institute of Ireland (RPII) – *www.epa.ie*

Duties of Employers and Employees

The **Safety, Health and Welfare at Work Act 2005** sets out the duties of employers and employees in Ireland.

Employers' Duties

The employer is responsible for ensuring, as far as is reasonably practicable, the safety, health and welfare at work of his or her employees. This includes providing:

- A safe place of work
- Safe systems of work
- Competent employees
- Safe equipment.

The employer must ensure that in the course of their work, employees are not exposed to risks to their safety, health or welfare.

> 'Every employer shall ensure, so far as is reasonably practicable, the safety, health and welfare at work of all his or her employees.'
>
> (Safety, Health and Welfare at Work Act 2005)

Sections 8 and 12 of the Act deal specifically with the duties of employers. The responsibility for safety and health management ultimately lies with the employer. This responsibility can be delegated within the organisation to directors, managers, etc., but the employer must ensure that the authority and duties of each individual are clearly communicated. The organisational and reporting structure for implementing these duties should be clearly illustrated in an in-house organisational chart, which should be included in the company's safety statement.

The Act states that, to prevent workplace injuries and ill health, every employer must:

1. Provide a safe place of work for employees, e.g. have enough space for staff to move around
2. Prevent any improper conduct and behaviour in the workplace likely to put the safety, health and welfare of the employee at risk

3. Provide a safe system of work and provide personal protective equipment (PPE), e.g. gloves and aprons
4. Provide safe access to and egress from the place of work
5. Provide adequate welfare facilities, e.g. toilets, washrooms, canteen, first aid station
6. Provide safe plant and equipment, e.g. hoist, oxygen cylinders
7. Check that equipment is properly used and regularly checked and maintained
8. Prepare adequate plans for employees to follow in emergencies, e.g. fire drills
9. Provide adequate supervision, e.g. nurse or manager in charge
10. Ensure competence by providing information (using language that can be understood by all) to instruct and train employees, e.g. on manual handling, safe use of sharps
11. Identify all hazards in the workplace, e.g. hazards that might cause back injury, stress
12. Conduct a risk assessment on all hazards identified and ensure appropriate control measures are put in place to eliminate the hazard or reduce the risk of the hazard; and report accidents to the HSA
13. Implement training and safe practice programmes, e.g. manual handling and client transfer training
14. Ensure compliance with relevant statuary provisions
15. Appoint a competent person as the organisation's safety officer
16. Create and make available a safety statement for the workplace.

Employees' Duties

Employees' legal duties are laid out in **Sections 13 and 14 of the Safety, Health and Welfare at Work Act 2005**. Employees must:

1. Take responsibility and reasonable care for their own safety, health and welfare and that of others who may be affected by their actions
2. Adhere to safe systems of work by using equipment in a safe manner, e.g. hoists
3. Not be under the influence of an intoxicant (e.g. alcohol, cocaine) in the workplace
4. Not engage in improper conduct or behaviour that will endanger themselves or others
5. Report defects, contraventions or danger in plant or machinery to their supervisor, e.g. equipment not working properly
6. Not intentionally interfere with safety equipment
7. Attend safety training provided by their employer and implement learning in the workplace
8. Comply with legislation and the organisation's safety statement
9. Make proper use of protective equipment, including PPE, and not interfere with, misuse or damage this equipment
10. Undergo any reasonable medical or other assessment if asked to do so by the employer.

These duties apply to all employees, including part-time and fixed-term employees, temporary and agency staff.

CHAPTER 01: HEALTH AND SAFETY LEGISLATION

Task

1. Read the following excerpt from Section 8 of the Safety, Health and Welfare at Work Act 2005.

   [A]n employer's duty extends to: ... managing and conducting work activities in such a way as to prevent any improper conduct or behaviour likely to put the safety, health or welfare at work of his or her employees at risk ... preparing and revising adequate plans and procedures to be followed and measures to be taken in the case of an emergency or serious or imminent danger ... reporting accidents and dangerous occurrences.

   (a) Consider why these provisions are included in the Act.

   (b) How effective do you think they are in reducing accident rates at work?

   (c) Discuss how each of these three duties may be performed by an employer in a healthcare facility.

2. Read the following excerpt from Section 10 of the Act:

   Every employer shall ... ensure that instruction, training and supervision is provided in a form, manner and language that is reasonably likely to be understood by the employee.

   (a) Why is this provision in the Act?

   (b) Discuss the difficulties of performing this duty in, say, a large hospital.

   (c) Consider the implications of this law in an organisation employing workers of many different nationalities.

The Safety Statement

The safety statement is a written document that outlines how safety, health and welfare is managed in the workplace. **Section 20 of the Safety, Health and Welfare at Work Act 2005** requires that an organisation produce this statement to safeguard the safety and health of:

+ Employees while at work

+ Other people who might be at the workplace, including service users, customers, visitors and members of the public.

Functions of the Safety Statement

The safety statement:

1. Specifies how health and safety will be managed within the workplace
2. Is the cornerstone of effective health and safety management
3. Contains policy and risk assessments
4. Outlines the controls required to minimise risks from hazards in the workplace
5. Details the names of those responsible for putting the controls into practice.

A safety statement specifies hazards identified in the workplace, based on risks assessed, and identifies the controls and resources that are in place to avoid or manage these risks. For example, a risk assessment may identify aggressive behaviour from residents as a risk factor. It will identify who could be harmed and how to establish any preventable measures already in place. The employer will then assess the risk and decide if more needs to be done to protect the employee and the other residents.

(HSA 2019a)

A safety statement should include all information relating to the relevant safety and health legislation, such as:

+ Details of how the safety and health of all employees will be secured and managed

- All occupational hazards and risks assessed
- A record of what is being done to prevent injury or harm to employees and others in the workplace, the protective and preventive measures taken, and the resources provided for safety and health at the workplace
- The employer's commitment to comply with legal obligations
- Information on how the employer will consult with employees on health and safety matters
- Plans and procedures to deal with emergencies
- The names, job titles and responsibilities of the employees with particular health and safety responsibilities in the workplace
- The duties of employees as required by law
- A review mechanism.

All information is to be written in a form, manner and language that will be understood by all.

The safety statement should be signed by the responsible person (e.g. employer/senior manager) and dated. It must be brought to the attention of:

- All staff and others at the workplace who may be exposed to the risks to which the safety statement applies
- Newly recruited employees on commencement of employment
- All staff members, if there has been any change in policy or work practice.

The employer must review the safety statement annually and change it if:

- There have been changes to policy or work practices affecting safety and health at work

- The employer believes that the safety statement is no longer valid

- An inspector dictates that the statement must be amended.

It is important that the organisation's safety statement is a living document, reviewed periodically and as work conditions change. It should always be prepared in consultation with employees and the written document brought to the attention of all workers and those who may be exposed to the risks to which the safety statement applies.

Preparing a safety statement will not prevent accidents and ill health at work, but by reflecting a commitment to promoting health and safety in the workplace and communicating the arrangements put in place, the safety statement will play a vital part in maintaining a safe, healthy and productive workplace.

Activity

True or False Quiz

1. A safety statement includes a client's care plan. True or false?

2. A safety statement is only for managers. True or false?

3. A safety statement must be brought to the attention of employees: when they start work; at least annually; and whenever the safety statement is amended. True or false?

4. A safety statement is based on the identification of work-related hazards and the assessment of the risks presented by those hazards. True or false?

Answers to quiz can be found on page 179.

chapter 2
A SAFE AND HEALTHY WORK ENVIRONMENT

IN THIS CHAPTER YOU WILL LEARN ABOUT:

- Factors that contribute to a safe and healthy working environment
- Principles and procedures of good housekeeping in the workplace
- Causes and prevention of accidents and dangerous occurrences, and emergency procedures to be followed
- Reporting and recording accidents to the relevant bodies

Workplace health relates to the effects of work on people's health and vice versa.

(HSA 2016a)

Work, if managed properly, is generally good for a person's physical and mental health; so a worker's environment should protect and promote their health.

According to the World Health Organization:

> [A] healthy workplace is one in which workers and managers collaborate to use a continual improvement process to protect and promote the health, safety and well-being of all

> workers and the sustainability of the workplace by considering the following, based on identified needs:
> - Health and safety concerns in the physical work environment.
> - Health, safety, and well-being concerns in the psychosocial work environment, including organization of work and workplace culture.
>
> (WHO 2010a)

Healthcare Injury Statistics in Ireland

In 2018, the healthcare sector accounted for 19.1 per cent of all workplace injuries reported to the HSA. The top three accident triggers were:

- Manual handling
- Slips, trips and falls
- Aggression, shock, fright or violence.

Reported incidents in the healthcare sector 2018

Cause	Number of incidents	Percentage
Manual handling	516	29.4
Aggression, shock, fright or violence	344	19.6
Fall on same level (slip, stumble, etc.)	333	19

(HSA 2019a)

In 2017, the Central Statistics Office (CSO) recorded the following:

- The illness rate for the healthcare sector was 42 per 1,000. The rate for all sectors was 28.

- The injury rate for the healthcare sector was 26 per 1,000. The rate for all sectors was 23.

(HSA 2019a)

Maintaining a Safe and Healthy Work Environment

To ensure a consistently safe and healthy work environment, it is vital that all staff take ownership of responsibility for safe practices and are aware of potential risks and hazards. Factors contributing to a safe and healthy work environment can be classed as:

- **Active actions:** good housekeeping, recognising and preparing for work-related risks and hazards
- **Reactive actions:** responding to, reporting and learning from accidents or incidents.

Active Monitoring

Active monitoring procedures monitor the design, development, installation and operation of safety systems and workplace precautions. The achievement of specific objectives and the extent of compliance to standards can be determined and essential feedback on performance can be provided. Active monitoring is undertaken *before* things go wrong, with routine inspections and checks carried out to see that standards are being maintained.

Active monitoring involves inspections and monitoring.

1. **Inspections:**
    - Formal/informal, planned /unplanned
    - Actual performance versus predetermined standard
    - Use of checklists.

2. **Monitoring:**
    - Environmental monitoring
    - Health surveillance
    - Audits
    - Independent review of the whole system.

An inspection system provides a basis for measuring achievement and identifying whether standards are being met. When introducing an inspection system, it is important that the following elements are addressed: events such as accidents, ill health, incidents and other areas of deficient health and safety performance.

Reactive Monitoring

Reactive monitoring is carried out after things go wrong by investigating injuries, cases of illness, bullying complaints, property damage and near misses, specifying in each case why performance was sub-standard.

Good Housekeeping

Effective housekeeping can eliminate some workplace hazards and prevent accidents. Good housekeeping means, for example, ensuring that corridors, work areas and floors are completely free from slip and trip hazards.

Good housekeeping implies that a workplace is kept in an organised, uncluttered and hazard-free condition. While this may seem a simple concept, good housekeeping practices can positively affect workers' safety, health and productivity.

Good housekeeping is not just about cleanliness; it also lays the foundation for accident and fire prevention. It requires attention to

CHAPTER 02: A SAFE AND HEALTHY WORK ENVIRONMENT

details, such as the layout or accessibility of the workplace; identifying and marking physical hazards; ensuring that there are an adequate number of storage facilities; and carrying out routine maintenance.

The Five Ss principle outlines how to achieve and maintain good housekeeping standards.

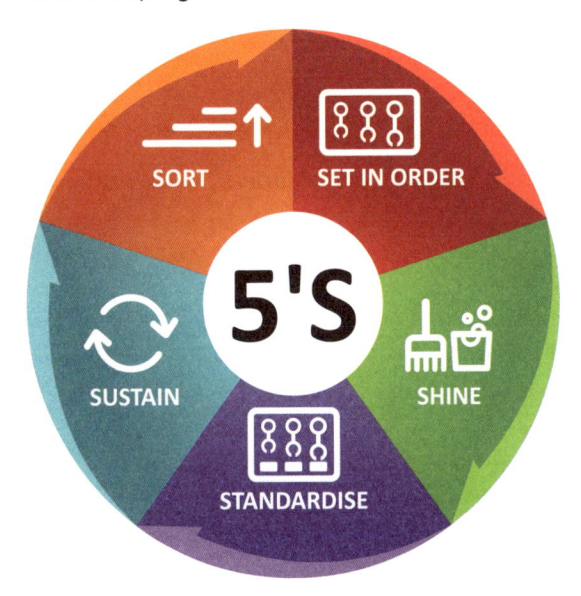

The Five Ss of good housekeeping.

1. **Sort:** Sort out unnecessary items in the workplace and discard them
2. **Set in order:** Arrange necessary items in good order
3. **Shine:** Clean the workplace thoroughly, leaving no dust on desks, floors, machines or equipment
4. **Standardise:** Maintain high standards of housekeeping at the workplace at all times
5. **Sustain:** Train people to follow good housekeeping rules.

(Hirano, Hiroyuki (1998) *Putting 5S to Work: A Practical Step-by-Step Approach.* PHP Institute of America)

Good Housekeeping Procedures

Good housekeeping standards are key to preventing accidents in busy work environments. A 'see it, sort it and tidy as you go' culture should always prevail among all staff; tidying up should not be left until the end of a shift.

Good housekeeping can be achieved by ensuring the following:

- Regular cleaning programmes
- Proper disposal of waste in accordance with national requirements
- Regular inspections of workshop areas and offices
- Identification of potential fire hazards, e.g. storing flammable liquids near potential heat sources
- A 'clean and tidy as you go' policy.

Good housekeeping procedures to prevent slips, trips and falls:

- Keep all walkways clear from obstructions.
- Provide bins and ensure that waste is removed regularly and appropriately.
- Provide and maintain adequate storage space and avoid clutter.
- Clean floors at quiet times when there is the minimum pedestrian traffic.
- Cordon off the floor area being cleaned using a barrier and provide dry paths through/around areas being cleaned.
- When wet cleaning, use water at the right temperature and detergent in line with manufacturer's instructions. Remove excess liquid to assist the floor drying process.

CHAPTER 02: A SAFE AND HEALTHY WORK ENVIRONMENT

- Ensure all cleaning staff have received adequate training, instruction and demonstrations.

- Ensure that personal protective equipment (PPE) is supplied based on risk assessment, e.g. slip-resistant footwear.

- Warning signs:

    - should be in place, but be aware that they do not substitute for necessary protective measures, e.g. warning signs do not keep people away from wet floors

    - may not be adequate for many circumstances and should only be used where hazards cannot be avoided or adequately reduced by other means

    - must be removed when they no longer apply. Always consider the use of the premises, its occupancy, the services being supplied and the activity that is taking place.

(HSE 2015)

Task Looking at the photograph, identify the hazards for staff and outline how staff could improve their housekeeping skills and procedures.

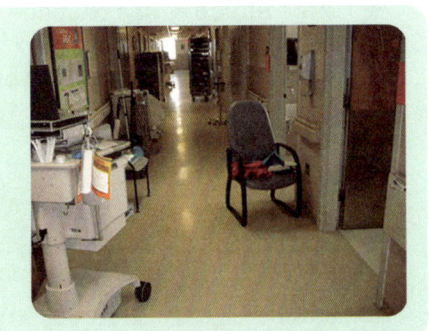

Benefits of Good Housekeeping

Effective housekeeping results in:

- Reduced handling of materials, which speeds up the flow of materials
- Fewer tripping and slipping incidents in clutter-free and spill-free work areas
- Fewer fire hazards
- Decreased exposure of workers to hazardous products (e.g. dusts, vapours)
- Better control of tools and materials, including inventory and supplies
- More efficient equipment clean-up and maintenance
- More hygienic conditions, leading to improved health
- More effective use of space
- Reduced property damage by improving preventive maintenance
- Less janitorial work
- Higher morale
- Improved productivity (equipment and materials will be easy to find).

Accidents and Incidents

An *accident* is an unplanned event that causes personal injury or damage to a client, property or the environment. An *incident* is an unplanned event that could have but did not cause injury or damage. The causes can be determined and controlled.

CHAPTER 02: A SAFE AND HEALTHY WORK ENVIRONMENT

According to the Health and Safety Authority (HSA 2016a), most workplace incidents are preventable. The healthcare sector reports approximately 1,400 injuries each year to the HSA, accounting for nearly 20 per cent of all workplace injuries reported to the HSA each year.

Reported incidents indicate three main accident triggers in the healthcare sector:

- Manual handling (client handling and handling of inanimate loads)
- Slips, trips and falls (on the level)
- Work-related shock, fright and violence.

Accidents and incidents can be prevented by:

- Conducting risk assessments
- Providing adequate training
- Adequate supervision
- Maintaining all equipment in good working order
- Ensuring all repairs to equipment are carried out by competent persons
- Communication and consultation with employees
- Employees reporting any defects they see in their place of work.

Emergency Plans

It is an employer's duty to have adequate plans in place to be followed by employees in case of an emergency. All employees should be made aware of the emergency plans and procedures.

The objectives of emergency plans are:

- To contain and control incidents to minimise their effects, and to limit damage to human health, the environment and property

- To implement measures necessary to protect human health and the environment from the effects of major accidents

- To communicate the necessary information to the public and to the services or authorities concerned in the area

- To provide for the restoration and clean-up of the environment following a major accident.

(www.hsa.ie)

Emergency Preparedness and Response

Pre-planning is essential to enable people to act to prevent disaster. It will also highlight any deficiencies or lack of resources, which can then be addressed before an actual emergency occurs. The plan should be familiar to all, outline clear roles and responsibilities and be regularly reviewed and rehearsed.

An emergency plan should include details of:

- Suitable warning and alarm systems
- Emergency scenarios and how to respond to them
- Emergency procedures in the organisation
- Key personnel and their responsibilities
- Emergency services
- Internal and external communication plan
- Training plans.

The emergency plan should be aligned with the workplace safety statement as required by **Section 20 of the 2005 Act**.
(NIFAST 2015)

It is mandatory for all employees to attend fire drill education sessions. Fire drills should be held regularly to ensure that all employees are aware of the procedures to follow.

Recording and Reporting

The workplace must have a policy in place that all employees and any others working on the premises report to the person in charge any work-related accident, incident or near-miss event, without unreasonable delay.

There are several reasons for having reporting procedures in place.

1. It ensures that any person suffering injury or ill health can be attended to

2. It allows the workplace or activity to be made safe and prevent recurrence

3. It allows the facts of the incident to be established and recorded in the event of any legal proceedings and determines whether any further reporting is required

4. It is a legal requirement that certain work-related accidents and dangerous occurrences are reported to the HSA

5. When an employee is absent for three consecutive days or more (not including the date of the accident) due to an injury sustained during their employment, the incident must be reported to the HSA.

(HSE 2015)

Under the **Safety, Health and Welfare at Work (General Application) Regulations 2016**, all employers and self-employed persons are legally obliged to report the injury of an employee as a result of an accident while at work.

According to the **Safety, Health and Welfare at Work (Reporting of Accidents and Dangerous Occurrences) Regulations 2016**, the following key points must be adhered to in the reporting of accidents and dangerous occurrences:

- Only fatal and non-fatal injuries are reportable. Diseases, occupational illnesses or any impairments of mental condition are not reportable.
- Fatal accidents must be reported immediately to the HSA or Gardaí. Subsequently, the formal report should be submitted to the HSA within five working days of the death.
- Non-fatal accidents or dangerous occurrences should be reported to the HSA within ten working days of the event.
- The injury of any employee, as a result of an accident while at work, that results in the employee being unable to carry out their normal work duties for more than three consecutive days, excluding the day of the accident, must be reported.

The **Safety, Health and Welfare at Work Act 2005** contains the following definitions:

- **Accident** means an accident arising out of or in the course of employment which, in the case of a person carrying out work, results in personal injury.
- **Personal injury** includes:
  - any injury, disease, disability, occupational illness or any impairment of physical or mental condition, and
  - any death, that is attributable to work.

Making the Report

Employers and the self-employed all have a duty to report accidents and dangerous occurrences to the HSA. Reports can be made online at www.hsa.ie.

Keeping Records

Those who are required to report accidents and dangerous occurrences under the Regulations are also required to keep records for a period of ten years from the date of the incident. Records can be kept in the same format as the report made to the HSA – a copy of the report submitted to the HSA will suffice.

For further information, read the HSA's guidance booklet (HSA 2016a), available on its website (www.hsa.ie).

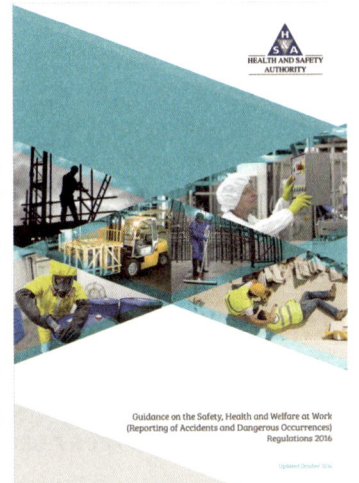

Reporting Accidents

All workplace accidents should be reported to the work supervisor and a record of the accident should be kept in the accident book/incident book in the workplace in accordance with local policy.

In line with the **Safety, Health and Welfare at Work (Reporting of Accidents and Dangerous Occurrences) Regulations 2016** (S.I. No. 370 of 2016), employers must report the following incidents to the HSA:

1. Any workplace accidents to employees that result in absence from work for three or more consecutive days following the accident, e.g. broken finger, back injury.

2. Specified dangerous occurrences, for example where an incident occurs but an employee is not injured, e.g. a chemical spillage in radiology, a fire in a building that results in the building being out of operation for 24 hours or more.

3. Specified occupational diseases, e.g. occupational deafness, mesothelioma (cancer of the lungs caused by exposure to asbestos), hepatitis B.

4. An accident causing the death of an employed or self-employed person.

5. An accident caused by a work activity that causes the death of, or requires medical treatment to, a person not at work, e.g. a visitor.

These accidents can be reported to the HSA via their online form.

It is essential that all internal reporting requirements are known to employees. Employees need to know:

- What needs to be reported
- Who makes the report
- Which report form is used
- Who the completed form goes to
- Who investigates.

Accident Investigations

The primary purpose of an accident investigation is to prevent accidents, not to apportion blame. An accident investigation should address the following elements:

- Identify failures in the safety management system
- Assist in preventing recurrences by enabling organisations to learn

- Satisfy legal recording and reporting requirements
- Collect information that may be needed if there is legal action
- Collect information for potential insurance claims.

It is important to make the distinction between a workplace accident and a healthcare incident and to whom each event should be reported. A workplace accident is an employee accident and must be reported to the HSA. However, if a client is involved in an accident, e.g. a fall, this must be reported to the Health Information and Quality Authority (HIQA).

See Appendix 1 for a sample accident/incident report.

Task 1

Recording and Reporting

Betty is a home care worker. On Tuesday she arrives, as scheduled, at her client Joan's house. Joan says that today she wants a bath instead of a shower. Joan's care plan states that she has showers because she has limited mobility to climb in and out of the bath, and her shower has been recently upgraded to a wet room. Betty explains to Joan that she should have a shower because it would be safer; and that she is not allowed to assist Joan in having a bath as it is not in her care plan. Joan becomes very angry and tells Betty to leave – she says that she will do what she wants and doesn't want anyone coming into her house telling her what to do. Betty tries to calm Joan down, but without success. She stands outside the front door, hoping that Joan will calm down and let her back in. After five minutes, Betty hears a loud noise from inside the house and Joan shouting 'Help, help!'.

1. Did Betty handle the situation well?
2. What should she do now?
3. What should Betty record regarding the incident?
4. When should she report the incident?

Task 2 — Writing an Accident Report

Give an example of a fall that might occur in a healthcare setting. Now write a report describing the environment, the client and their actions, the accident, the outcome of the fall and actions taken afterwards.

1. Was this an accident or an incident?
2. Who should fill in the report form?
3. What date and time should be included?
4. What location should be included?
5. Who should write the assessment for the fall?

chapter 3
RISK ASSESSMENT

IN THIS CHAPTER YOU WILL LEARN ABOUT:

- Risk assessments in the workplace
- The difference between a hazard and a risk
- Control measures
- How to perform a risk assessment
- Lone workers
- Night/shift workers

As we learned in Chapter 1, a safety statement is a written document that explains how an employer intends to protect the safety and health of their employees and others who may be affected by activities in the workplace. The safety statement includes risk assessments and a written commitment to managing safety and health in the workplace.

What is a Risk Assessment?

Section 19 of the Safety, Health and Welfare at Work Act 2005 requires that employers and those who control workplaces must identify the hazards in the workplaces under their control and assess the risks to safety and health at work presented by these hazards.

Risk assessment is the cornerstone to providing a safe and healthy working environment, and **Section 19 of the Act** requires every employer to identify workplace **hazards** and assess the **risk** associated with each hazard.

A risk assessment involves examining what, in the workplace, could cause harm to people and whether or not there are enough precautions in place to prevent it. It involves identifying hazards (anything that can cause harm) and risks (the likelihood of someone being harmed by the hazard and how severe the harm might be). The employer has the responsibility to take steps to implement any improvements considered necessary to guarantee the health and safety of all employees.

> A **hazard** is anything with the potential to cause harm in terms of human injury or ill health, such as work materials, equipment, work methods or practices, poor work design or exposure to harmful agents such as chemicals, noise or vibration.
>
> A **risk** is the likelihood that somebody will be harmed by the hazard and how serious the harm might be. When considering risk, you should also consider the number of people at risk from the hazard and their profile.
>
> **Chance** (or likelihood) is a measure of how likely it is that an accident could happen. When people are working safely there is less chance that an accident will occur.
>
> **Severity** is a measure of how serious an injury or damage to health as a result of unsafe working could be and is influenced by: the environment; the number of people at risk; and the steps already taken to control the hazard.
>
> **Control measures** (or controls) are the precautions taken to ensure that a hazard will not injure anyone. A control measure must not create an additional hazard.

The HSA explains the difference between risks and hazards as follows:

> If there was a spill of water in a room then that water would present a slipping hazard to persons passing through it. If access to that area was prevented by a physical barrier then the hazard would remain though the risk would be minimised.
>
> (HSA 2016a)

Assessing risk means that anything in the workplace that could cause harm to employees and other people (including customers, visitors and members of the public) must be carefully examined to estimate the level of risk and decide whether the risk is acceptable or whether more precautions are needed to prevent harm.

Employers are required to implement any improvements considered necessary by the risk assessment. However, it is important to remember that, in identifying hazards and assessing risks, employers should only consider those that are generated by work activities. There is no need to consider every minor hazard or risk that we accept as part of our lives.

The results of any risk assessments must be written into the safety statement.

Why Perform a Risk Assessment?

The main aim is to make sure that no one gets hurt or becomes ill. Accidents and ill health can ruin lives and can also negatively affect business. The main reasons for performing risk assessments are:

1. **It's the law:** Under the **Safety, Health and Welfare at Work Act 2005** an employer is required to carry out risk assessments, prepare a safety statement and implement what it contains. HSA inspectors visiting workplaces or investigating accidents will scrutinise the risk assessment and safety statement, and the procedures and work practices in operation. If any one of these is inadequate, the employer will be required to revise it. Employers can be prosecuted if they do not have a safety statement.

2. **It's good business:** A safe and healthy workplace contributes to an efficient business. Costs associated with accidents and ill health in the workplace can be significant and can include:

    - Salary costs for replacement staff or overtime payments
    - Lost productivity
    - Compensation pay-outs
    - Retraining costs
    - Increased insurance payments.

   Work-related diseases and ill health result in more than one million lost working days every year. These cases are due to failures in workplace safety and health management and can be extremely costly to a business and to the economy.

3. **It's the ethical thing to do:** The consequences of a workplace injury or illness can be long-lasting and devastating, both for the victim and for their family and loved ones. Employers have an ethical duty to do their best to prevent this, by providing a safe working environment for employees, allowing them to return home unharmed after each working day.

Performing a Risk Assessment

The **Health, Safety and Welfare at Work Act 2005** identifies five steps to follow to complete a risk assessment:

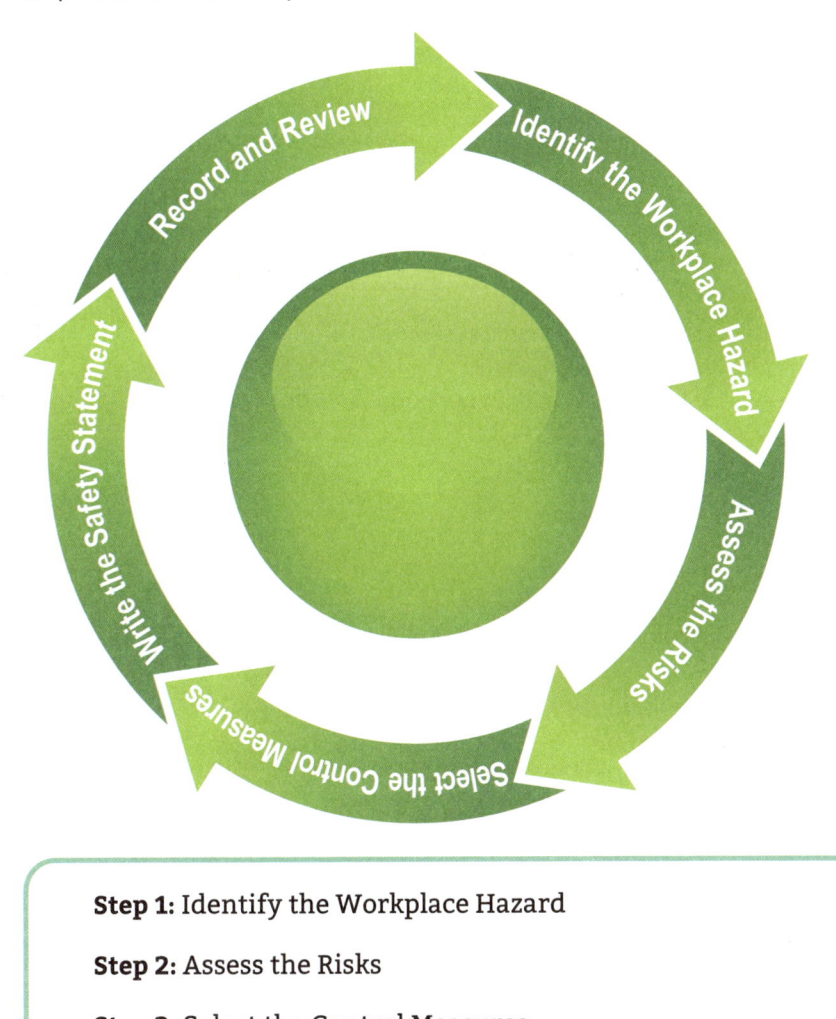

Step 1: Identify the Workplace Hazard

Step 2: Assess the Risks

Step 3: Select the Control Measures

Step 4: Write the Safety Statement

Step 5: Record and Review

Step 1: Identify the Workplace Hazard

A hazard is anything with the potential to cause injury or ill health. In any workplace there may be several different types of hazard:

- **Physical hazards**, such as:
    - manual handling (back injury)
    - slip or trip hazards (wet floor, no signage, uneven floor covering)
    - poor housekeeping (untidy corridors, misuse of equipment, non-compliance with systems of work)
    - fire (fire exit not clear, non-compliance with fire regulations, lack of training)
    - working at height
    - working with hot items
    - working in cold environments
    - ergonomics and display screen equipment (DSE)
    - driving for work or using poorly maintained equipment

- **Health hazards**, such as:
    - noise (a high level of noise over a sustained period can contribute to occupational deafness)
    - vibration
    - electricity (faulty electrical wiring or electrical equipment)
    - unsuitable light levels
    - harmful dusts

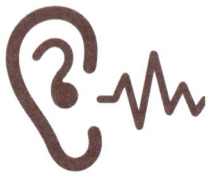

- stress
- waste disposal (needles in clinical waste)
- infection control (contract biological/viral infection)

+ **Chemical hazards**, such as:
    - working with common everyday products such as cleaning agents
    - glues and corrosive fluids, industrial solvents
    - dyes
    - radiation
    - biological agents
    - pesticides or acids

+ **Human factor hazards**, such as:
    - bullying
    - violence from other employees or members of the public.

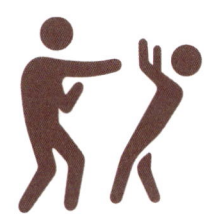

Some hazards are obvious, but it is important to be aware of the less obvious hazards such as excessive noise or exposure to chemicals, where it could take months or even years before ill health materialises.

Once you have identified the hazards, you can start to assess the risks.

Step 2: Assess the Risks

A risk is the likelihood of harm occurring and the severity of the consequences if it does.

Risk also depends on the number of people who might be exposed to the hazard.

In assessing the risk, you should estimate:

- How likely it is that a hazard will cause harm
- How serious that harm is likely to be
- How often and how many workers are exposed.

To quantify the level of risk that the hazard will pose, the risk of the hazard must be categorised as low, medium or high. For example, a needle-stick injury in an emergency department may create a high risk and if dealt with incorrectly can lead to serious injury.

- **Low risk:** The likelihood of an accident occurring is low and the severity is low, e.g. intermittent work on a computer where the workstation is well laid out is unlikely to result in any harm to the user.

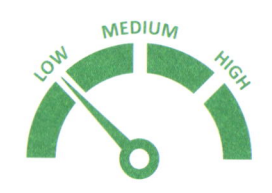

- **Medium risk:** As the levels of likelihood and severity increase, a hazard may be assessed as a medium risk, e.g. manual handling of heavy loads without mechanical aids.

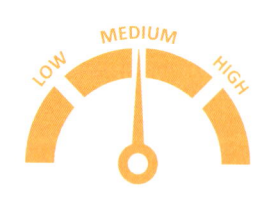

- **High risk:** There is a likelihood that an accident could occur and if it does there could be serious injuries, ill health or death, e.g. vehicles reversing where pedestrians or members of the public are walking.

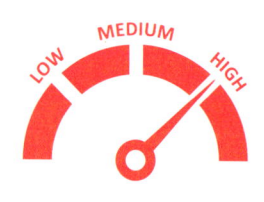

    High-risk hazards should be focussed on first.

When assessing the risk, it is important to consider who may be exposed to a specific hazard. Direct employees, contract staff (such as cleaners, outside maintenance personnel) and visitors should be included in your assessment.

Risk is normally assessed by using a matrix such as this:

		Impact				
		Very Low	Low	Medium	High	Very High
Probability	Very Likely	allow	mitigate	avoid	avoid	avoid
	Likely	accept	allow	mitigate	avoid	avoid
	Possible	accept	allow	allow	mitigate	avoid
	Unlikely	accept	accept	allow	allow	mitigate
	Rare	accept	accept	accept	accept	allow

Step 3: Select the Control Measures

A **control measure** is any action that can be taken to:

+ Reduce the potential of exposure to the hazard

+ Remove the hazard

+ Reduce the likelihood of exposure to the hazard being realised.

(HSA 2016a)

It is important to note that eliminating a risk is not always possible, and in these circumstances a control measure that reduces the risk of injury to an absolute minimum should be chosen. Examples of control measures are: providing a hoist and providing sharps bins to reduce the risk of needle-stick injuries.

Control measures are often organised into a hierarchy with the most preferred control measures at the top of the triangle and less preferred measures at the bottom.

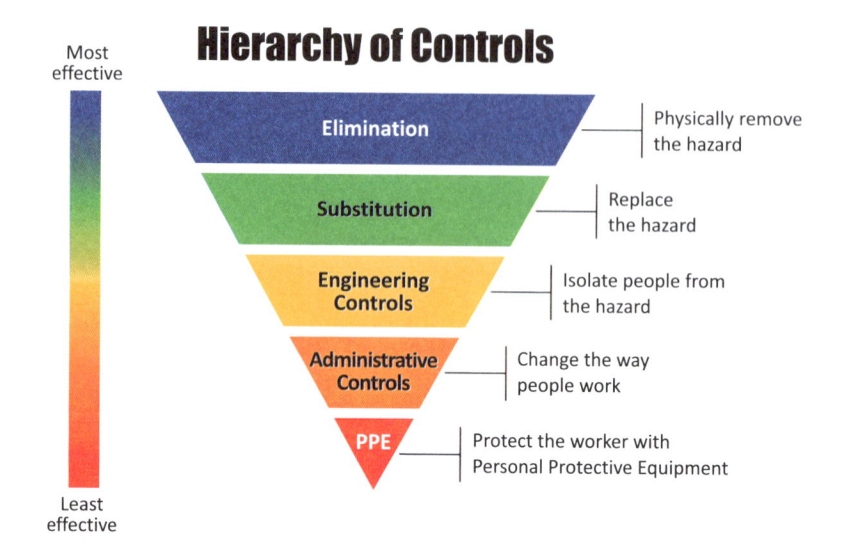

Hierarchy of Controls

Most effective → Least effective:
- **Elimination** — Physically remove the hazard
- **Substitution** — Replace the hazard
- **Engineering Controls** — Isolate people from the hazard
- **Administrative Controls** — Change the way people work
- **PPE** — Protect the worker with Personal Protective Equipment

(2015 National Institute for Occupational Safety and Health. https://www.cdc.gov/niosh/topics/hierarchy/default.html)

Hierarchy of Control

+ **Elimination**

    Where possible, eliminate the hazard completely.

    Example: Second-hand smoke. Eliminate smoking in and around healthcare facilities.

+ **Substitution**

    Substitute the less dangerous for the dangerous. This may not remove all the hazards/hazardous activity and may introduce different hazards, but the overall harm or health effects will be reduced.

    Example: Scented products that may induce allergic reaction. Substitute with less harmful products or maintain adequate general ventilation.

✚ Isolation

Restrict access to the hazard or lock the hazard away under strict controls.

Example: Airborne biological agents contactable by secretions from infectious clients (coughing, sneezing, etc.). Early detection of infection status, followed by isolation and vaccines.

✚ Engineering controls

Redesign a process to place a barrier between the person and the hazard or remove the hazard from the person.

Example: Lifting clients. Introduce hoist lifts.

✚ Administrative controls

Develop a policy and ethos of accident prevention. Adopt standard operating procedures or safe work practices, or provide appropriate training.

Example: Manual handling training; sharps awareness training; isolation; permit-to-work procedures.

✚ Personal protective equipment (PPE)

PPE, including gloves, glasses, earmuffs, aprons, safety footwear, dust masks, are designed to reduce exposure to the hazard, helping to combat risk at source. PPE is usually seen as the last line of defence and is normally used in conjunction with one or more of the other control measures.

Example: It is widely recognised that single-use surgical masks cannot offer any real protection against small particles and may lead to a false sense of security, thereby increasing risk. The additional use of an extraction system with positive/

negative air flow and fitted respirators may be necessary where the hazard may have significant health effects.

Other common control measures include:

- Ensuring a clean and tidy workplace to prevent slips, trips and falls

- Adapting the work to the individual, e.g. providing adjustable-height tables or chairs

- Switching off and isolating machines before carrying out repairs or alterations

- Safeguarding machinery

- Establishing emergency procedures, including first aid

- Providing adequate training for workers

- Containing the hazard at source, e.g. providing local exhaust ventilation or a fume cupboard with extraction

- Ventilating the whole area of the workplace where extraction at source is not possible

- Providing protective equipment, clothing or signs (to be used only as a last resort after all other ways of controlling the hazard have been fully explored)

- Setting up adequate health surveillance programmes including pre-placement or regular health checks where appropriate

- Having appropriate policies in place, such as anti-bullying.

Audit

It is essential that the outcomes of the control measures introduced are audited to determine how well the aims set down are being achieved. Corrective action should be taken when required.

Step 4: Write the Safety Statement

Once the employer has completed steps 1–3, they must complete a safety statement.

A safety statement must include:

- Control measures to be taken to avoid the risks identified
- The names of those responsible for implementing and maintaining the control measures
- Contact details of key persons responsible in the event of an emergency
- Names of the safety representatives.

The safety statement should contain four sections:

- Section 1: Health and safety policy
- Section 2: Safety arrangements and information
- Section 3: Forms and records
- Section 4: Risk assessments and action list.

The safety statement must be reviewed annually, or if the work environment or practices change, or as and when a new risk is identified. Read Chapter 1 to recap on safety statements.

Step 5: Record and Review

The findings of the risk assessment process must be recorded. See Appendix 2 for an example of a completed risk assessment.

Employees must be informed of the control measures that have been put in place. Communicating with employees the risk assessment and its findings ensures that:

- Employees fully understand what is expected of them in working safely

- Employees know who is responsible for implementing any additional controls and by what date these controls must be put in place

- Employees are encouraged to monitor the effectiveness of the control measures in place and communicate with management if they feel additional control measures are required.

The following is an example of a risk assessment process in a healthcare environment.

1. Identification of the hazard – Needle-stick injury

2. Identification of who may be harmed – Client, nurse, healthcare assistant, housekeeping staff, ancillary staff

3. Assessment of the risk – High

4. Identification of control measures – PPE; adherence to policy, i.e. tray sharps disposal unit, education, audit practice

5. Record and review – Risk assessment documented and reviewed as per policy.

Task Complete a risk assessment on your college building and present a report on your findings.

See Appendix 2 for an example of a completed risk assessment form, and go to www.borupress.ie to download a blank template.

The risk assessments and safety statement should be brought to the attention of all employees and others in the workplace. As new employees are particularly at risk when starting a new job, they must be made aware of the safety statement when they start work.

Other people may also be exposed to a specific risk and they too should be made aware of the statement. These people may include:

- Outside contractors, cleaners, maintenance or building staff, or sub-contractors from another employer
- Temporary workers who are not familiar with your work
- Delivery people who come into contact with activities on your premises
- Self-employed people who provide a service to the employer.

Activity

You have been tasked with running an intergenerational dance class for residents, their families and friends in a nursing home. Your manager has requested that you complete an audit on the class to ensure that the building is safe, using the following guidelines:

1. Identify a comprehensive hazard identification.
2. Complete an evaluation of the risk associated with each hazard.
3. Identify control procedures for identified risks.
4. Do a re-evaluation of risks after implementation of control measures.
5. Make relevant recommendations.

Lone Workers

Lone workers are those who work alone at a place of work or in isolation at remote locations. The **Safety, Health and Welfare at Work Act 2005** and the **Safety, Health and Welfare at Work (General Application) Regulations 2007** take account of particular risks to this group.

Lone workers are at increased risk of violence and aggression at work, manual handling incidents and accident, and medical emergencies because they work alone, or because they are more likely to take risks and do not have the support of a colleague in, for example, assisting or supporting a client. It is incumbent on the employer to specifically manage safety, health and welfare at work for lone workers by identifying hazards, assessing risks, identifying controls and providing safe systems of work and safe equipment to avoid these risks.

A clear plan for emergencies must be made and appropriate information, training and supervision must also be provided. The lone worker must always feel supported and part of the wider healthcare setting.

Task

Consider the role of a lone worker visiting a client in their home. This client lives with a relative but is alone by day. He uses a walking frame as he has some mobility issues; he also has speech difficulties, making communication a challenge.

Conduct a risk assessment on a visit to this client's home.

Night Work and Shift Work

Shift work is common practice in healthcare work, and it is accepted that the majority of healthcare staff will do shift work at some stage in their career. While there are several reasons for the prevalence of shift work, such as business needs and the need to provide a 24-hour service, it must be acknowledged that there are negative health effects from this form of work.

There are several illnesses associated with night workers and shift workers, which are primarily due to disruption of the circadian rhythms, resulting in hormone imbalance (melatonin suppression), sleeping difficulties and fatigue. Chronic fatigue resulting from night and shift work is strongly associated with gastrointestinal illnesses such as abdominal pain, chronic gastritis and peptic ulcers, and cardiovascular illnesses such as hypertension and coronary heart disease.

(HSA 2012)

The effects of prolonged shift work include risk of errors and accidents in the workplace. Errors and accidents at work tend to:

- Be higher on night shifts
- Rise with increasing shift length over an eight-hour threshold
- Increase over successive shifts (especially night shifts)
- Increase when there are insufficient breaks due to poorly designed shift schedules; this results in fatigue, which in turn leads to poor performance, errors and accidents.

Legislation

The **Safety, Health and Welfare at Work (General Application) Regulations 2007, Chapter 3 of Part 6: Night Work and Shift Work**

> The Night Work and Shift Work Regulations impose duties on an employer in relation to employees who are defined as night workers and shift workers. These duties include carrying out a risk assessment and implementing protective measures for both night and shift workers; making available a health assessment and possible changes to working conditions and transfer to day work where a doctor is of the opinion that a night worker is, or could become, ill as a result of night work.
>
> (HSA 2012)

Younger Workers

While the employment of children under 16 years is generally prohibited by the **Protection of Young Persons (Employment) Act 1996**, a child over 14 years may be permitted to do light work during school holidays provided it is not harmful to health, development or schooling, or may be employed as part of an approved work experience or education programme. A child over 15 years may also do such work for up to eight hours a week during the school term. The Act also sets limits to the working hours of young persons (i.e. 16- to 17-year-olds), who may not work for more than eight hours in any day or 40 hours in any week.

> An employer must carry out a risk assessment before employing a child or young person and whenever there is a major change in the place of work, which could affect the safety or health of the child or young person.

The employer is required to carry out a risk assessment prior to a child or a young person commencing employment. Also, when there is a major change in the place of work or the work to be carried out, the employer is required to ensure that there is no significant risk to the safety and health of the child or young person.

An employer must assess any risk to the safety or health of a child or young person and any specific risk to their safety, health and development arising from

- his or her lack of experience, absence of awareness of existing or potential risks or lack of maturity
- any work activity likely to involve a risk of harmful exposure to the physical, biological and chemical agents
- the processes and work

and take the necessary preventive and protective measures.

The employer must ensure that any risks to the safety and health of a child or young person or to their development are assessed, taking into account the increased risk arising from the child's or young person's lack of maturity and experience in identifying risks to their own safety and health and, specifically, that any exposure to physical, biological and chemical agents or certain processes is avoided.

(Regulation 144: Risk Assessment as amended by the Safety, Health and Welfare at Work (General Application) (Amendment) Regulations 2007, HSA 2007)

Task: Younger Workers

Denise is 16 and recently applied for a part-time job as tea lady in the local nursing home. Denise wants to be a social care worker so she feels this will really suit her and give her experience for her future career.

Denise gets the job, and as it is part-time she will still be able to attend school and meet her friends. During school term she ends up working ten hours a week and once the summer holidays start she begins to get more hours as the other ladies who work there take holidays. Some weeks Denise ends up working 48 hours as she also covers the girl doing the washing-up in the kitchen. Sometimes on her tea rounds she is asked by carers to move residents from one chair to another.

1. What is the maximum number of hours Denise should be working during school term?

2. As a 16-year-old, is Denise allowed to work 48 hours a week?

3. Is Denise going beyond her duties when assisting carers?

4. Are there any safety and health issues in this scenario?

chapter 4
HAZARDS IN THE WORKPLACE

> **IN THIS CHAPTER YOU WILL LEARN ABOUT:**
> - Types of hazards in the workplace:
>   - physical
>   - chemical
>   - psychosocial
>   - biological
> - Healthcare waste (non-risk and risk)
> - Disposal of hazardous materials and waste in the workplace
> - Safety data sheets

> A workplace hazard can be described as any object, condition or practice that can cause injury.

When identifying a hazard, it is important to consider who might be harmed by the hazard and how, taking into account:

- The various categories of staff who may be exposed

- The service users and those who may infrequently visit the workplace, e.g. visitors, contractors, cleaning staff, members of the public, etc.

- Those who may be more vulnerable, such as pregnant women, people with different abilities or disabilities, new or inexperienced workers, workers whose first language is not English

- Lone workers, night workers and shift workers.

Hazards can have varying degrees of danger, depending on the person(s) who encounters them.

In the work environment, there are four types of hazard that can potentially threaten the health and safety of healthcare workers: physical hazards; chemical hazards; psychosocial hazards; and biological hazards.

Physical Hazards

- Manual handling activities involving heavy, awkward or hard-to-reach loads
- Machine-related injuries from equipment that has been poorly maintained, is used incorrectly or is not suitable for the task
- Electrical dangers
- Ergonomic-related risks (repetitive motion, awkward posture, using excessive force)
- Radiation exposure
- People's behaviour and physical attributes. A positive attitude to health and safety by all in the workplace will create a safer working environment. Taking account of physical disabilities such as poor vision, limited mobility etc. in planning and design will help reduce the risk
- Slipping and tripping on wet or poorly maintained floors, or over mats or other items left on the floor.

Specific considerations for floors include:

- Floor surface – must be suitable for the work activity and kept in good condition

CHAPTER 04: HAZARDS IN THE WORKPLACE

- Floor contamination and obstacles – prevent contamination (wet floors, greasy floors, paper wrappers, etc.) and improve housekeeping and the risk will be reduced if not eliminated
- Floor cleaning – stop pedestrian access to wet floors; spot clean where possible
- Environmental aspects – ensure adequate lighting for walkways and level changes; good entrance design (e.g. canopies) can help
- Footwear – wearing suitable footwear for the environment and work activities will help reduce the risk.

As a healthcare assistant, a potential hazard that you must constantly be aware of on a day-to-day basis is the risk of slips, trips and falls. In healthcare, the risk of slips, trips and falls is high as the people being cared for are often vulnerable due to poor health, have limited mobility and may have physical disabilities. The health condition of the client must be considered when assessing the environment for potential risks from slips, trips and fall hazards.

Here are some examples of physical hazard areas within the healthcare environment:

- Stairs and steps are a potential hazard for both staff and clients.
- Crash mats: while a crash mat prevents the client from having a hard fall to the ground from the bed, it can present as a hazard for staff when working around the bed area.

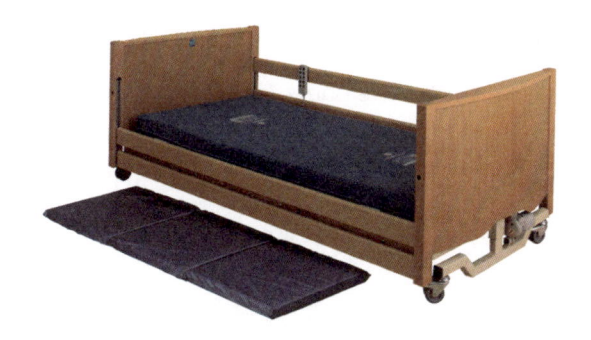

These hazards must be recognised, assessed, minimised, eliminated or controlled.

Chemical Hazards

Chemical use is widespread in many workplaces and especially so in the healthcare sector. Chemicals used include:

- Cleaning agents
- Disinfecting and sterilising agents
- Laboratory chemicals
- Medical gases
- Anaesthetic agents
- Cytotoxic drugs and pharmaceutical substances.

Any chemical that has the potential to cause harm is called a hazardous or dangerous chemical. Hazardous chemicals can have many negative effects, including:

- Health effects such as a respiratory effect or skin irritant
- Physical hazards from a flammable, explosive or oxidising chemical
- Environmental impact, if chemicals are used, stored or disposed of incorrectly.

Healthcare workers may suffer health effects when dangerous chemicals enter the body. The main routes of exposure are:

- **Inhalation:** breathing in the chemical
- **Absorption:** through skin contact or a splash in the eye

- **Ingestion:** via contaminated food or hands
- **Inoculation:** when a sharp object such as a needle punctures the skin.

The **Safety, Health and Welfare at Work (Chemical Agents) Regulations 2001** and the **Safety, Health and Welfare at Work (Carcinogens) Regulations 2019** require that employers must assess any work activity likely to involve a risk of exposure to chemicals, carcinogens or mutagens. Employers should also have emergency plans and procedures in the event of an uncontrolled release, leak or spillage of a dangerous chemical.

Psychosocial Hazards

Psychosocial hazards include violence at work and work-related stress.

> These stresses can be harmful to the mental and physical health of healthcare workers, with evidence of two to three times greater risk of mental illness, injuries, back pain, and workplace conflict and violence.
>
> (Stoewen 2016)

Violence at Work

Work-related violence and aggression has been defined by the European Commission as any incident where staff are abused, threatened, or assaulted in circumstances related to their work, involving an explicit or implicit challenge to their safety, well-being or health.

(EASHW 2011)

What Constitutes a Violent Act?

An aggressive or violent act can be physical, such as spitting, using force against a person, such as pushing, hitting or punching, or attacking a person with a weapon or object; or non-physical, such as verbal abuse, threats or gestures.

Violence and aggression can be considered a potential hazard in the healthcare sector and must be risk-assessed. Where there is a risk to health and safety from violence, appropriate safeguards must be put in place. Employers' duty to identify the hazards in their workplace, assess the risks to employees and put in place appropriate control measures applies to the issue of violence and aggression at work as much as any other work-related hazard.

Preventing Violence at Work

Prevention of harm or violence at work takes place at two levels:

1. Preventing acts of violence occurring, or reducing them by identifying hazards, assessing risks and taking preventive action where necessary. Staff training on how to deal with violent clients is also essential.

2. If an act of violence occurs, support is required for the person who has experienced the incident to minimise its harmful effects.

The Effects of Violence at Work

The consequences for the individual vary depending on the context in which violence occurs and the personal characteristics of the victim. The effects can include:

- Injury to physical or psychological health
- Demotivation

CHAPTER 04: HAZARDS IN THE WORKPLACE

- Reduced pride in performing one's job
- Stress (even for an indirect victim, the witness of the violent act or incident)
- Post-traumatic symptoms such as fear, phobias and sleeping difficulties
- Post-traumatic stress disorder (PTSD).

In cases of physical violence, the evidence is quite easy to establish. It is harder, however, to determine the reaction or effects of repeated acts of psychological violence.

Violence also has an impact on the organisation because people who work in an environment of fear and resentment cannot give their best. The negative effects on the organisation will be reflected in increased absenteeism, decreasing motivation and reduced professionalism.

Task: Violence at Work

Alli has recently started work in a new nursing home where there is an 18-bed dementia unit. Alli has never worked with people who have dementia, so she has no experience of their behaviours, and she made this clear to the employer at the beginning of her employment. She is told that she will shadow other carers in the unit to learn the process of how it works, and she will receive both dementia training and responding to challenging behaviour training over the next two months.

Three months have now passed and Alli shadowed one carer in the dementia unit for six hours but so far has received no training. The nursing home is short-staffed and Alli is asked to go into the dementia unit to cover lunch. Alli is in the unit with one other carer and a nurse and lets them know she was only in there briefly once before. She is asked by the nurse to take John to the toilet as he is walking around the halls opening his trousers. Alli asks John if he wants to go to the toilet. John does not respond to her question, so she begins to guide him to the bathroom. Once they get to the bathroom John begins to shout at Alli and is not making sense. She becomes fearful and asks John to assist her by sitting on the toilet. John gets angry, hits out at Alli and strikes her in the stomach. Alli goes back out to tell the nurse what happened, and the nurse tells her not to worry – she will be okay.

1. How did the employer fail to provide a safe working place for Alli?
2. What could the employer have implemented to safeguard Alli?
3. How do you think this act of violence will affect Alli in her work in the future?
4. What would have made Alli's experience better?

Work-related Stress

Work-related stress among employees in Ireland doubled between 2010 and 2015. In 2015, 17 per cent of the workforce experienced stress, up from 8 per cent in 2010; however, the Irish figure of 17 per cent was still below the European average of 19 per cent. Workers most likely to report stress were in the health sector (18 per cent), while employees exposed to bullying, harassment and violence were eight times more likely to be stressed than those in jobs with no such exposure.

(ESRI 2015)

Employees experience work-related stress when the demands of the work environment exceed the employees' ability to cope with (or control) them. Stress is not a disease, but if it is intense and goes on for some time, it can lead to mental and physical ill health.

Work-related stress can be caused by psychosocial hazards, such as work design, organisation and management, and issues such as bullying and violence at work; or physical hazards, such as noise and temperature.

The causes of work-related stress can be many and varied but can be broadly classified into three groups.

1. Stress from doing the job: caused by monotonous work, too much work or insufficient time to do the work.

2. Stress from work relationships: due to poor teamwork, complex hierarchies of authority, working in isolation or bullying and harassment.

3. Stress from working conditions: shift work, dealing with life-threatening injuries, illnesses and client deaths or the threat of violence and aggression.

Work-related stress is preventable and the risk assessment for stress involves the same basic principles and process as for other workplace hazards. The involvement of workers and their representatives in the risk assessment is crucial to its success; they should be asked what is causing stress, which groups are suffering and what could be done to help.

(EASHW 2002; HSE 2018)

Symptoms of stress and anxiety include:

1. Taking more time off work than usual

2. Greater use of substances such as alcohol, tobacco and drugs (prescription and illegal)

3. Increased irritability, poor concentration, reduced productivity

4. Deteriorating personal or work relationships, including bullying behaviours

5. Becoming more 'emotional', moody or over-reactive to what others say

6. Starting to behave differently/exhibiting behaviour that is 'out of the norm'

7. Changing of eating and sleep patterns

8. Physical reactions such as sweating, palpitations and increased blood pressure

9. Feeling negative, depressed and anxious most of the time

10. Feeling trapped or frustrated and believing there's no solution.

(Hughes 2013)

Biological Hazards

Exposure to biological hazards in healthcare may be:

+ Intentional, through working with biological agents in a laboratory setting, or

+ Unintentional, through client care activities where the exposure may accidentally arise as a result of the type of work being carried out.

(HSA website: 'Biological Agents')

Healthcare workers may come into contact with several sources of infection through direct contact with clients who have infections or with contaminated materials, such as waste, laundry or contaminated surfaces.

The **Safety, Health and Welfare at Work (Biological Agents) Regulations 2013 (S.I. No. 572 of 2013)** and the related Code of Practice set down the minimum requirements for the protection of workers from the health risks associated with biological agents in the workplace. The HSA is the enforcing agency with regard to these regulations.

Healthcare Waste

Healthcare waste is the solid or liquid waste arising from healthcare and can be either non-risk waste or risk waste. The majority is non-risk domestic waste and can be carefully disposed of as household waste.

Non-risk Waste

This can be categorised as domestic waste, and includes:

1. Normal household and catering waste that cannot be recycled. It is all waste that is non-infectious, non-toxic, non-radioactive and non-chemical. Examples include general everyday items like food waste and packaging.

2. Medical equipment that is assessed as non-infectious, which means it has not been contaminated by blood or body fluids. Items in this category include oxygen face masks, empty urine catheter drainage bags, empty enteric feed bags and disposable gloves and aprons.

3. Potentially offensive material, including incontinence wear from non-infected clients and stoma bags that have not been soiled with blood. This material is deemed non-infectious.

4. Confidential material, including shredded waste and confidential documents.

Risk Waste

Healthcare risk waste is potentially hazardous and carries a risk of being infectious to those who come into contact with it. It contains used sharp materials that could cause injury. The Department of Health and Children's 'Segregation, Packaging and Storage Guidelines for Healthcare Risk Waste' defines potentially offensive infectious waste and outlines the precautions to be taken when handling and storing risk waste.

(DoHC 2004)

Risk waste can include general risk waste, chemical risk waste and sharps.

- General risk waste includes:
  - blood and items that are soiled with blood, e.g. dressings, swabs, bandages, gloves and aprons
  - incontinence wear from clients who have a known or suspected enteric infection, e.g. *Salmonella*, *Clostridium difficile (C.diff)* or Norovirus
  - items contaminated with body fluids other than faeces, urine or breast milk.
- Chemical healthcare risk waste includes discarded chemicals and medicines.
- Sharps are any object that has been used in the treatment of a client and are likely to cause a puncture wound or cut to the skin, e.g. syringes, needles, scalpels and razor blades.

Disposal of Healthcare Risk Waste

There are several different types of risk waste bags and boxes used in the healthcare setting, both acute and community. All bins are coloured yellow with colour-coded lids for different uses.

A yellow bag is used for blood-stained or contaminated items which are soft, e.g. soiled dressings, swabs bandages, gloves and incontinence waste for clients that are known or suspected to have an enteric infection.

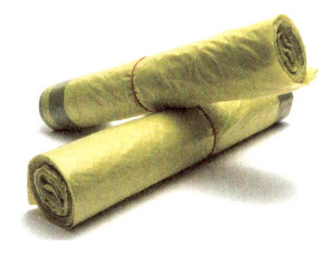

CHAPTER 04: HAZARDS IN THE WORKPLACE

A yellow rigid box with a yellow lid is used to dispose of contained body fluids and blood, e.g. vacuum dressing suction machine liners, dialysis equipment and sputum containers.

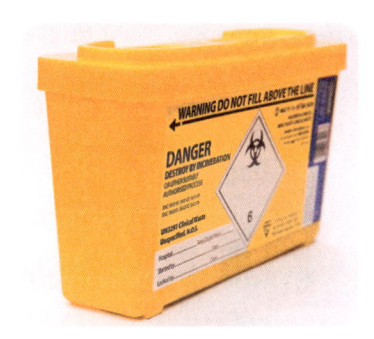

A yellow rigid box with a purple lid is used to dispose of chemicals and medicines from pharmacy.

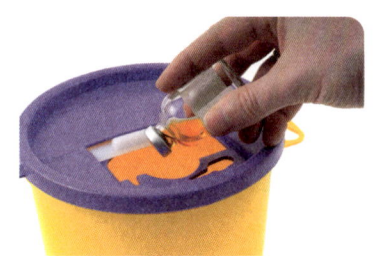

A yellow sharps bin with a blue or red lid should be used for sharp items such as needles, syringes, scalpels and stitch cutters.

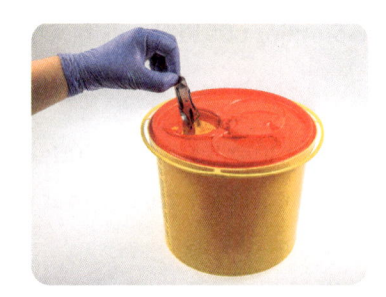

A yellow sharps bin with a purple lid is used to dispose of sharps that have been used to administer cytotoxic drugs such as intravenous sets, needles and syringes.

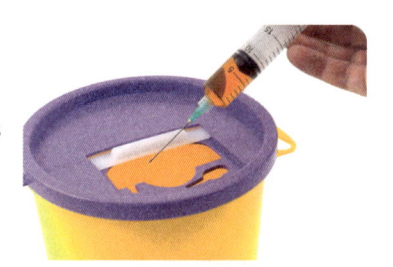

Biohazard bags are for bloodstained or contaminated items, including dressings, swabs and bandages from infected clients and PPE (gloves, aprons and gowns) used by staff members when attending to infected clients.

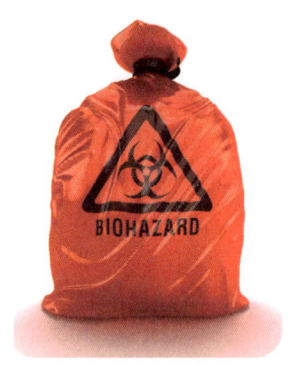

These materials must be disposed of as follows:

- All items to be placed in yellow biohazard bag – do not overfill.
- Bags must be securely closed with a cable tie or tape when two-thirds full maximum.
- When securely tied, the bags must be removed to the designated area.
- Bags must not be used for sharp or breakable items or for liquids.

Sharps

Sharps are 'any object which has been used in the diagnosis, treatment, or prevention of disease that is likely to cause a puncture wound or cut to the skin'.

(DoHC 2000)

Sharps injuries can include puncture of the skin by a needle, syringe, broken glass or razors that have become contaminated by blood from infected clients.

Guidance for Handling Sharps

- Avoid the use of sharps if possible.
- All staff who handle sharps should be immunised against hepatitis B.
- Sharps containers must comply with **National Standards (UN 3291, BS 7320)**.
- Sharps containers must be assembled correctly with an identification label.
- Sharps containers should be available at the point of use.

- When transporting a used syringe (e.g. arterial blood sampling), remove the needle using a removable device and attach a blind hub prior to transportation.

- Avoid re-sheathing needles manually and re-sheath as a last resort.

- To re-sheath safely, place the sheath on a flat surface. Only re-sheath needles if a device is available to allow this to be done using one hand only.

- Do not pass sharps from hand to hand; use a kidney dish/tray.

- When using sharps during a procedure, ensure that they do not become obscured by dressings, paper towelling, drapes, etc.

- Always provide assistance to a nurse or doctor when they are taking blood/giving injections to unco-operative or confused clients.

Safe Disposal of Sharps

- Inspect refuse bags before removal/transport in case of inappropriate disposal of sharps.

- Never discard needles/syringes/sharps in a polythene bag.

- Discard sharps at the point of use into a sharps container and immediately following use.

- Discard disposable syringes and needles wherever possible as a single unit, into the sharps container.

- Sharps such as small quantities of broken glass, drug vials, used needles, razor blades, etc. must be carefully disposed of into approved sharps containers.

- Never attempt to decant the contents of small sharps containers into larger containers.

- Never dispose of sharps in containers used for storage of other wastes, or place used sharps containers into clinical waste bags.

- Never leave sharps lying around.

- Never insert fingers/hand below the level of the lid.

- Close the aperture on the disposal container of each sharp at the client's bedside.

- Ensure the sharps containers are free from protruding sharps.

- Sharps containers should not be filled above the fill line. Replace when three-quarters full.

- Once full, the container aperture must be locked, tagged and identification label signed.

- The person locking the sharps container must tag the sharps container.

Needle-stick Injury Procedure

If a healthcare worker receives a needle-stick injury, the following procedure must be followed:

- Squeeze the wound to encourage bleeding.

- Wash the wound under cold running water.

- Cover the wound with a dressing.

- Report the injury to management.

- Post exposure, the staff member must be tested for hepatitis B, hepatitis C and HIV.

- Monitor and re-test the affected staff member for blood-borne pathogens after a six-week period and again at six months.

HSE (2012) *Patient Safety Toolbox Talks*

Remember!

- **Bleed it**
- **Wash it**
- **Cover it**
- **Report it**

Safety Data Sheet (SDS)

The appropriate procedure for the use and disposal of hazardous materials and waste in the workplace is determined by the recommendations issued by the manufacturer of the chemical/hazardous material, which will comply with European and national laws and regulations. The most important reference point relating to procedure for the use and disposal of hazardous materials and waste is the **safety data sheet** (SDS).

The SDS is a document that contains information on the potential hazards (health, fire, reactivity and environmental) of a chemical product (e.g. sulphuric acid, Parazone disinfectant) and how to work safely with the product. It contains information on correct use, storage, handling and emergency procedures. The SDS contains much more information about the material than the label.

An SDS is prepared by the supplier or manufacturer of the material. It is intended to identify the hazards of the product, inform how to use the product safely, what to expect if the recommendations are not followed, what to do if accidents occur, how to recognise symptoms of overexposure, and what to do if such incidents occur.

All SDSs have 16 sections and each numbered section must refer to a specific heading as detailed below:

- **Section 1: Identification of the substance/mixture** and of the company/undertaking to include product identifier; relevant identified uses of the substance or mixture and uses advised against; details of the supplier of the SDS; emergency telephone number

- **Section 2: Hazards identification,** e.g. classification of the substance or mixture

- **Section 3: Composition/information on ingredients,** i.e. substances used in manufacture

- **Section 4: First aid measures**

- **Section 5: Firefighting measures,** e.g. extinguishing methods

- **Section 6: Accidental release measures,** e.g. personal precautions, protective equipment, emergency procedures

- **Section 7: Handling and storage,** e.g. precautions for safe handling

- **Section 8: Exposure controls/personal protection,** e.g. control parameters

- **Section 9: Physical and chemical properties**

- **Section 10: Stability and reactivity,** e.g. possibility of hazardous reactions

- **Section 11: Toxicological information**

- **Section 12: Ecological information,** e.g. mobility in soil

- **Section 13: Disposal considerations,** e.g. waste treatment methods

- **Section 14: Transport information,** e.g. transport hazard class(es)

CHAPTER 04: HAZARDS IN THE WORKPLACE

- **Section 15: Regulatory information** e.g. safety, health and environmental regulations/legislation specific to the substance or mixture

- **Section 16: Other information:** any other relevant information.

> **Task**
> 1. Select a household product, for example a cleaning agent. Search online for the product's SDS. **Tip:** search for the supplier's name; from their website you should be able to get a copy of the SDS.
> 2. Discuss your findings in class.

chapter 5
OCCUPATIONAL HEALTH RISKS

IN THIS CHAPTER YOU WILL LEARN ABOUT:

- A range of occupational health issues
- How these health issues affect the health and safety of workers
- Control measures to consider for these health risks
- Specific hazards and risks when working with equipment, including mechanical and electrical equipment

Common health and safety issues in healthcare include noise, fumes and dust, dangers to the skin, manual handling and misuse of/faulty equipment.

Noise

Occupational noise exposure can lead to temporary hearing loss, sometimes followed by permanent hearing loss. The two factors that cause occupational noise-induced hearing loss are:

1. The noise level, measured in decibels (dB/dBA)
2. The duration of exposure to the noise level.

Noise, in its different manifestations, can have profound impacts on staff, residents and visitors in healthcare facilities, ranging from soothing and therapeutic to stressful and disturbing. Joseph and Ulrich (2007) found that hospitals are extremely noisy, and noise levels in most hospitals far exceed recommended guidelines. High ambient noise levels, as well as peak noise levels in hospitals, have serious impacts on client and staff outcomes, ranging from sleep loss and elevated blood pressure among clients to emotional exhaustion and burnout among staff.

A poorly designed acoustic environment can pose a serious threat to client confidentiality if private conversations between clients and staff or between staff members can be overheard by unintended listeners.

Noise Control

Noise meters can measure noise levels, and, if required, risk assessment must be undertaken where workers are subjected to excessive noise levels in the workplace, i.e. 80 dBA or greater. If levels are too high, steps must be taken to bring the levels within acceptable parameters to avoid unnecessary negative health effects to workers, clients or visitors.

Fumes and Dust

Fume and dust exposure in the workplace can lead to a range of health problems associated with both the inhalation of and contact with the dust or fumes.

The types of fumes and dust that healthcare workers may come into contact with include cleaning and disinfectant agents, latex from gloves, dusty storage rooms and clients' or residents' second-hand smoke.

Control measures for fumes include face masks, adequate ventilation and reducing exposure to the specific cause of the problem.

Asthma

Occupational asthma is asthma that is caused by breathing in chemical fumes, gases, dust or other substances while at work. It can also result from exposure to a substance that one is sensitive to, causing an allergic or immunological response. Like other types of asthma, occupational asthma can cause chest tightness, wheezing and shortness of breath. Healthcare workers with allergies or with a family history of allergies are more likely to develop occupational asthma.

(Mayo Clinic 2019)

When an asthma attack occurs, the muscles surrounding the airways become tight and the lining of the air passages swells, reducing the amount of air that can pass by, possibly leading to wheezing sounds. Asthma attacks can last minutes to days and can become dangerous if the airflow becomes severely restricted.

Work-related asthma accounts for about 10 per cent of all adult onset asthma. Asthma related to the workplace can be categorised into two distinct subsets: work-aggravated asthma and occupational asthma.

Allergic occupational asthma is caused by sensitisation or becoming allergic to a specific chemical agent in the workplace over a period of time and it accounts for over 90 per cent of cases of occupational asthma.

(HSA 2008)

Preventing and Controlling Occupational Asthma

Once a risk assessment has been completed and it has been identified that workers are being exposed to respiratory sensitisers, the following control measures should be considered:

- Stop using the sensitiser by replacing with a safer alternative if available.

- Segregate the work so as to minimise the number of workers exposed.
- Totally enclose the process, if possible.
- If this is not possible, partially enclose the process and provide local exhaust ventilation.
- If after carrying out these control measures there is still exposure, provide suitable personal respiratory protection to workers.

(HSA 2008)

Protecting the Skin

The skin is the largest organ in the body. Protecting the skin from workplace hazards is a priority to reduce the risk of vocation-specific hazards to employees. Hand, eye, head and body protection are used to protect the employee from a range of hazards. Skin contact with workplace dust, fumes, chemicals and spillages can lead to a range of skin conditions including dermatitis, eczema, burns and ulceration.

Use of Gloves

Appropriate use of gloves (latex or non-latex) is essential. Completing a risk assessment on the individual employee will clarify the appropriate PPE to use. However, it is important to note that latex in many medical products can itself pose a health problem to those with latex allergy.

Natural rubber latex (NRL) is used in medical gloves and many other medical products, such as elasticised bandages, dressings, etc., and it can cause asthma and dermatitis. Allergy to certain latex proteins emerged as an occupational disease in the 1980s and as NRL products are used increasingly worldwide, particularly in healthcare, it continues to be a significant occupational health problem. The use of gloves is an important element of infection prevention and control in healthcare and cannot be eliminated in the regime to protect the healthcare workers from hazards.

Effects of latex allergy symptoms range from a rash, itchy or runny eyes or nose, sneezing and coughing to chest tightness, shortness of breath and anaphylactic shock. The symptoms experienced depend in part on the route of exposure, which can be by direct contact with skin or mucosa, or by inhalation.

Types of allergic reaction to latex

Type	Signs/ symptoms	Cause	Comment
Irritant contact dermatitis	Scaling, drying, cracking of skin	Irritation by gloves, powder, soaps/ detergent, incomplete hand drying	Most common reaction to glove use
Allergic contact dermatitis, type IV delayed hypersensitivity, allergic contact sensitivity	Blistering, itching, crusting	Processing chemicals	Appearance like that of poison ivy rash

Type	Signs/symptoms	Cause	Comment
Immediate hypersensitivity, IgE/histamine-mediated allergy, type I hypersensitivity	Local: hives Systemic: generalised urticaria, rhinitis, wheezing, asthma, swelling of mouth, shortness of breath, can lead to anaphylactic shock	Latex proteins – direct contact or inhalation	Anaphylactic shock is very rare and is treated with adrenalin

(HSA (2001) Report of the Advisory Committee on Health Services, Dublin)

Hand Washing

Hand washing is one of the most important tasks that a healthcare worker can perform to protect the client from the spread of infection.

In healthcare there are two methods for effective hand washing:

+ Soap and water
+ Alcohol hand rub.

Both methods may contribute to development of dermatitis or eczema if not conducted appropriately, so ongoing training in methodology and aftercare is essential to reduce these side effects.

Case Study

Christina is a healthcare worker employed full time in the HSE. She works in the accident and emergency department of University Hospital Limerick. This department can become very loud and busy during peak times, due to the high numbers of people attending with different types of illness. As part of Christina's job description, she must clean down the wheelchairs and beds with disinfectant after each use.

Task Carry out a risk assessment of Christina's job, documenting the risk of noise, fumes and occupational-related injury and listing essential controls for these risks.

Manual Handling

Manual handling is the highest accident trigger reported to the Health and Safety Authority (HSA) by the healthcare sector. In 2018, 516 incidents, 29.4 per cent of the total number of incidents reported by the healthcare sector to the HSA, were manual handling incidents. These incidents concern both client handling and the manual handling of inanimate loads. The most common cause of reported incidents was lifting or carrying.

(HSA 2019a)

The **Safety, Health and Welfare at Work (General Application) Regulations 2007, Chapter 4 of Part 2 (S.I. No. 299 of 2007)**, also known as the **Manual Handling of Loads Regulation**, outlines the requirements that must be fulfilled in relation to manual handling. Manual handling of loads as defined in the Regulation includes any lifting, putting down, pushing, pulling, carrying or moving of a load which, by reason of its characteristics or unfavourable ergonomic conditions, involves risk, particularly of back injury, to employees. The basic principle enshrined in Part 2 is that where manual handling of loads involving a risk of injury (particularly to the back) is present, the employer must take measures to avoid or reduce the risk of injury.

Key requirements in this regulation are:

1. Avoidance of manual handling activities that involve a risk of injury

2. Risk assessment of manual handling tasks that cannot be avoided

3. Reduction of the risk from manual handling activities.

Manual Handling Risk Assessment

A manual handling risk assessment can fall into the following categories:

- **Generic ward/department risk assessment:** An assessment of the general situation usually found in the ward or department, taking account of the work environment and how the work is organised in relation to manual handling.

- **Task-specific risk assessment:** Where the ward/department level risk assessment identifies that a manual handling activity presents a risk of injury, the activity must be assessed in greater detail to determine what controls are required.

- **Individual client handling risk assessment:** Where a client cannot move independently and manual handling by the employee is needed, an individual client risk assessment will be required (preferably at admission), resulting in a handling/mobility care plan for the client.

Manual handling risk assessments should be conducted by a person with the necessary competence and training. In doing so, risk factors detailed in **Schedule 3 of the Safety, Health and Welfare at Work (General Application) Regulations 2007** (see Appendix 2) must be considered. These risk factors are summarised with the acronym TILE:

+ **T**ask: requirements of the activity such as excessive lifting, lowering or carrying distances, physical effort which may be too strenuous, etc.

+ **I**ndividual: the individual's physical capability, training and knowledge

+ **L**oad: the characteristics of a load – which can be either an object or a person – such as weight, size, difficulty of grasping, etc.

+ **E**nvironment: available space, uneven or slippery floors, unsuitable temperature, etc.

(HSE 2011, p. 189)

The overall approach to risk management should be outlined in the healthcare setting's manual handling policy and included in its safety statement.

Once the risk factors relating to the environment and the individuals carrying out the activity have been identified, the required controls must be decided. Controls may include team handling involving two or more carers and/or manual handling equipment to reduce the degree of manual handling required. When manual handling equipment is identified as a control measure, information about the equipment, such as the type and size of sling required, should be specific.

If handling with more than one person is required, good communication is essential: the leader should be nominated and agreed and words of command clarified.

Risk assessments and care plans must be reviewed and revised if necessary (e.g. if the client's condition improves/deteriorates and this affects the type of assistance required, or if on review the controls are shown not to be effective).

Risk assessment forms and care plans for client handling activities should be clear and well laid out and should be easily accessible to any staff who require them.

> **Task:** What type of injury could a healthcare worker acquire if they do not use the hoist correctly?

Mechanical Equipment

Working with any type of equipment presents its own set of work-related hazards. All hazards (anything that has the potential to cause harm) in the workplace must be risk-assessed, which involves identifying the hazard and assessing the risk (likelihood of an undesired event occurring).

Using mechanical equipment can put the employee at risk of injury. Training and adherence to policy and standard operating procedures will reduce risk of injury. To minimise the risk to staff working in healthcare, it is of vital importance that employers are aware of the manual handling regulation contained in the **Safety, Health and Welfare at Work Act 2005**.

The hazards associated with mechanical equipment include:

+ **Noise:** can potentially lead to deafness
+ **Vibration:** hand/arm vibration and whole-body vibration can cause harm to joints

- **Moving mechanical components/parts:** potential to cause injury, e.g. back injury
- **Fire:** burns, inhalation damage
- **Dust:** asthma
- **Fumes and vapours:** poison, toxicity
- **Crush:** fracture or fatal injury.

Appropriate risk assessment will identify these hazards, assess the risk and identify appropriate controls to eliminate or reduce the risk to workers.

Some of the mechanical equipment that may be used in a healthcare setting are mechanical beds, hoists, client handling aids and medical appliances.

Electrical Equipment

Electricity can cause direct and indirect harm. Direct harm is when electricity passes through the body, which can cause convulsions, make the heart stop beating and either internal or external burns. Any one of these or a combination can kill. Indirect harm caused by electricity can cause small electric shocks to lead to other accidents, e.g. overheating equipment can cause fire; short circuits can lead to equipment damage.

Electrical equipment hazards include:

- Electrocution
- Fire
- Electrical short circuit
- Electrical arcing

- Electrical burns
- Working in damp or wet conditions
- Working in confined spaces.

These hazards can result in injuries such as smoke inhalation and burns or in death.

Simple Electrical Safety Rules

- Ensure electrical equipment is suitable for the working environment.
- Connect all equipment to fixed mains sockets, where possible.
- Ensure that all socket circuits are protected by a residual current device (RCD).
- Test the RCD regularly.
- Avoid the use of extension leads and multiple adaptors.
- Never swap equipment leads between devices.
- Have a recorded inspection and maintenance programme for all electrical equipment.
- Train staff to carry out visual inspections for damage (such as exposed wires and scorching on plugs, leads and cables) and report faults.
- Take faulty equipment out of use immediately until repaired. Clearly label as faulty or remove the plug to prevent use.
- Never clean or adjust appliances when the power is switched on.
- Never touch light switches or appliances with wet hands.

(HSA website)

chapter 6
FIRE PREVENTION

> **IN THIS CHAPTER YOU WILL LEARN ABOUT:**
> - Fire prevention
> - Fire detection and warning
> - Fire triangle
> - Ignition sources
> - Preventing the spread of fire
> - Emergency escape and firefighting
> - Personal emergency evacuation plan (PEEP)

Fire prevention is a vital issue in the safety, health and welfare of everyone working within a healthcare setting. It is essential that all staff are aware of how to prevent fire and know the procedure of the safe evacuation of clients, visitors and employees if fire does break out.

In Ireland, the primary legislation governing fire safety in buildings to which the public are admitted is the **Fire Services Act 1981** and **2003**. This legislation places a duty of care on every person who has control over a premises to take all reasonable measures to guard against the outbreak of fire on their premises and to ensure as far as is reasonably practicable the safety of persons on the premises in the event of an outbreak of fire.

The **Safety, Health and Welfare Act 2005** and the **Safety, Health and Welfare at Work Act 2007** also place a general duty of care on employers in respect of workplace health and safety. The Health and Safety Authority (HSA) has the authority to monitor risks associated with fire in the workplace, while local fire authorities have the power to give advice, issue recommendations and enforce compliance.

Employer and Employee Responsibilities in Fire Prevention

The **Safety, Health and Welfare at Work Act 2005** states that all employers must have adequate policies and procedures in place to deal with an emergency situation. **Section 11 of the 2005 Act** states that employers are required to prepare and revise adequate emergency plans and procedures and provide the necessary measures for fire-fighting and evacuating the workplace.

Employees must be trained in fire safety, and in all healthcare settings annual fire training is mandatory. Healthcare settings will have different policies, procedures and practices. Employers have a duty to bring these to the attention of all employees, and all staff must take personal responsibility for ensuring that they are fully aware of these policies and understand them clearly.

Section 12 of the 2005 Act clarifies that consideration must also be given to the safety of persons other than employees within the workplace. Everything reasonably practicable must be done to ensure that all individuals at the place of work are not exposed to risks to their safety and health.

(HSA website: 'Emergency Escape and Fire Fighting')

It is the duty of each employee to:

- Co-operate with their employer – take part in fire drills
- Take reasonable care for their own health and safety

- Take reasonable care of others who may be affected by their acts or omissions at work

- Not intentionally interfere with or misuse equipment, e.g. fire alarms and fire extinguishers.

Under **Section 19 of the 2005 Act**, employers are required to carry out risk assessments and to record these in the safety statement. A fire safety risk assessment should include:

1. Fire prevention

2. Fire detection and warning

3. Emergency escape and firefighting.

> The best way to deal with a fire is to prevent it!

The Fire Triangle

Fire events have many causes, including poor housekeeping, faulty electrical equipment, poor storage of flammable materials and carelessness with ignition sources, e.g. cigarettes, candles and matches. Fire can only occur when oxygen, heat and fuel are present in sufficient quantities

Oxygen, heat and fuel are frequently referred to as the 'fire triangle'. Add a fourth element – chemical reaction – and you have a 'fire tetrahedron'. The important thing to remember is that if you take any of these four things away you will not have a fire, or the fire will be extinguished. Essentially, fire extinguishers put out fire by taking away one or more elements of the fire triangle/tetrahedron.

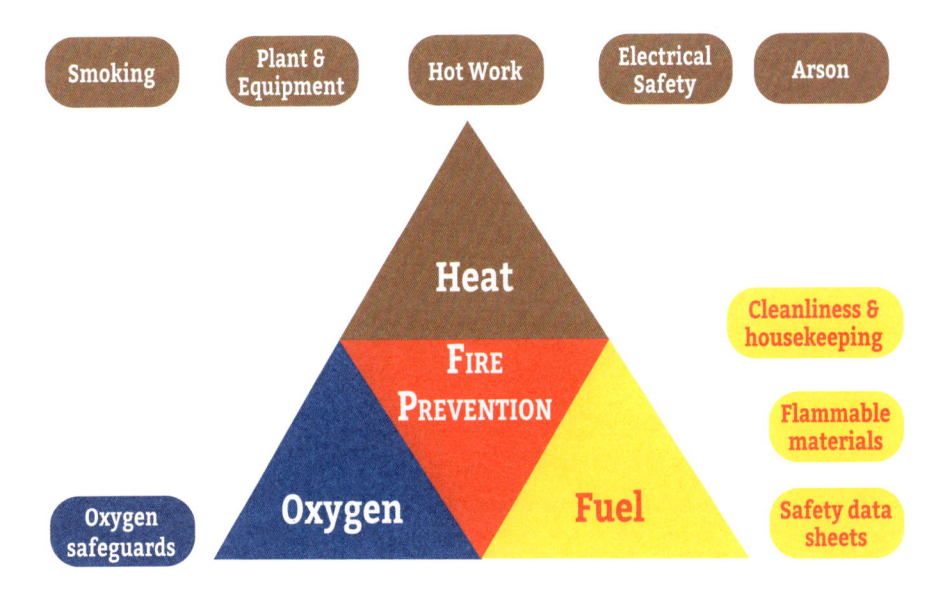

Ignition Sources

Fire safety, at its most basic, is based on the principle of keeping fuel sources and ignition sources separate.

Sources of potential ignition include sources of heat that may become hot enough to ignite material located close by. These sources include:

+ **Oxygen**, which is commonly used in healthcare facilities such as residential care centres. High concentrations of oxygen can cause materials to burn extremely rapidly and can cause some materials to burn that are not normally combustible. It can also cause an explosion if in contact with materials such as grease and oil. Smoking should not be allowed anywhere near areas where oxygen is used or stored. Storage areas must be labelled and risk assessments carried out.

(HSA 2019a)

+ **Smoking:** Careless use of cigarettes and other smoking materials is a common cause of fire in healthcare facilities. Staff need to be vigilant. A resident risk assessment must be completed, and controls put in place. Examples of controls are:

1. Sufficient ashtrays should be provided.

2. Ashtrays should not be emptied into plastic waste bags.

3. The number of combustibles in dedicated smoking rooms should be limited.

4. Inspections of smoking areas should be made regularly.

5. Protective bibs must be considered.

(HIQA 2016)

How Fire Spreads

Once started, a fire is likely to spread until all fuel has been used up, with possibly devastating consequences. By understanding how fire spreads, you may be better equipped to extinguish it.

Chemicals and combustibles: When fire comes into contact with lab chemicals, household cleaners, paint or any other chemicals, the fire burns hotter and more aggressively, causing it to spread. Other combustibles such as mattresses, sofa cushions, magazines, newspapers and various textiles will also have the same effect.

Open space: A building with limited interior structure burns much faster than one with hallways and closed doors. Walls and doors trap the fire and contain the flames and smoke. While the fire will eventually burn through the structure and continue to spread if left to its own devices, it is easier to control the flames in a building with more walls and doors, especially if those structures are built to withstand the heat and damage of a fire.

Construction materials: While a fire can burn through any building, those made of concrete and steel curb the spread of fire better than buildings made of timber frames.

Ventilation: Some buildings with central heating or air conditioning have ductwork, which can provide a way for flames and smoke to spread between floors of a building, even when the structure is primarily concrete and steel.

Water: In some cases, water is not a suitable fire extinguisher. Grease fires can spread faster when doused with water. A special fire extinguisher should be used to suffocate and stop the spread of grease fires in the kitchen.

Extinguishing a Fire

A fire will be put out if one of the three elements of the fire triangle is removed. This can be done using three different approaches:

1. **Cooling:** Removing heat is one of the most effective methods of fire extinction, which is why water is an effective extinguishing material. However, water is not appropriate for use on electrical fires or fires caused by cooking oils/fats or other flammable liquids.

2. **Starving:** While cooling removes the heat/ignition element of the fire triangle, starving the blaze of its fuel source is another approach. A raging fire will burn itself out if it runs out of flammable materials, for example a bonfire out in the open (not in contact with any other wood or dry grass) or a gas fire will immediately go out once the supply of material is gone.

3. **Smothering:** Removing oxygen from the equation is the final way of extinguishing a fire. Smothering a frying pan blaze with a fire blanket reduces the oxygen, similar to covering a candle with a glass. Smothering is a technique that is mostly applicable to solid fuel fires, although some materials may contain enough oxygen in their chemical make-up to keep the blaze burning.

> **Task**
>
> Rooms that pose a fire hazard include kitchens, bedrooms, laundries, switch rooms, boiler rooms, fuel storage areas, medical gas storage areas, stores, etc.
>
> In groups, discuss the hazards in these areas.

Fire-fighting Equipment

Fire Extinguishers

Fire extinguishers should be provided throughout all healthcare facilities. The type of fire extinguisher should be appropriate to the risk. They should be positioned on escape routes, close to rooms or storey exits and, if necessary, next to hazards. They should typically be placed on a stand or hung on a wall so that they can be easily accessed if required.

(HIQA 2016)

Trained professionals should check fire extinguishers and electrical equipment at prescribed intervals and evidence should be provided on the equipment of the date that testing took place.

(HSA 2019a)

Fire Extinguisher Operation

The guidelines for the correct use of a fire extinguisher are abbreviated as PASS:

+ **P**ull the pin
+ **A**im at base of fire
+ **S**queeze the handle
+ **S**weep extinguisher in a side to side motion

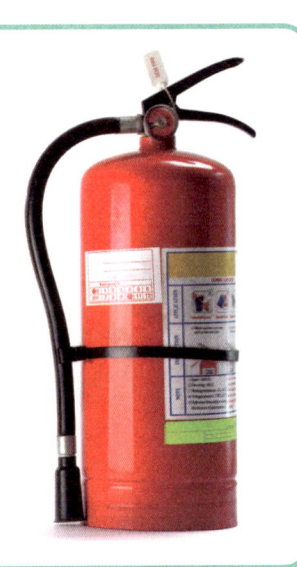

Safe Use of Fire Extinguishers

1. Raise the alarm
2. Do not tackle a fire alone, unless safe to do so
3. Choose the correct extinguisher
4. Remove safety devices
5. Test extinguisher to ensure it is working
6. Do not go too close to the fire
7. Keep low and watch for flare-ups
8. Do not let the fire cut off your escape route.

The type of fire determines which extinguisher should be used. Fires are classified as follows:

+ Class A – ordinary combustibles or solids, e.g. paper, wood
+ Class B – flammable or combustible liquids and liquefiable solids, e.g. paint, petrol

+ Class C – flammable gases and liquefied gases, e.g. butane, methane

+ Class D – combustible metals, e.g. lithium, potassium

+ Class E – electrical, e.g. computers, generators

+ Class F – cooking oils and fats, e.g. chip pans.

	Water	Dry Powder	Foam	Carbon Dioxide	Wet Chemical
A – Solids	✔	✔	✔	✘	✔
B – Liquids	✘	✔	✔	✔	✘
C – Gases	✘	✔	✘	✘	✘
D – Metals	✘	✘	✘	✘	✘
E – Electrical Hazards	✘	✔	✘	✔	✘
F – Fats/ Cooking Oils	✘	✘	✘	✘	✔

Important!

+ Tackling a fire with the incorrect extinguisher can lead to serious consequences. If in doubt, do not use an extinguisher.

+ Ensure the used extinguisher is set aside to be recharged.

Fire Blankets

A fire blanket smothers fire. It is suitable for using on burning clothing and small fires in contained vessels such as chip pans or deep fat fryers. The fire blanket removes all sources of additional oxygen and can only be used once.

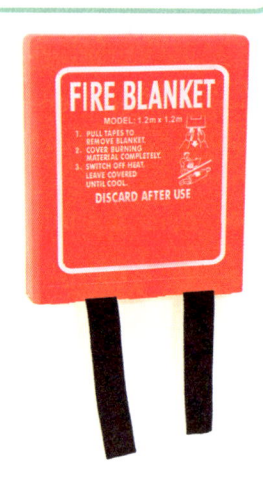

Stop-drop-roll is a simple fire safety technique used when a person's clothes are on fire: stop, drop, then roll the person in a fire blanket.

(HSE 2020)

Fire Evacuation Procedures

A fire evacuation plan must be drawn up and documented. It should take into account all the ways in which the building is used, look at all times of the day and night (day shift and night shift) and consider all users of the building.

All escape routes should be clear from obstruction and must be sufficiently wide (one metre) to enable evacuation of the building, considering the physical condition of residents and the evacuation methods likely to be employed. The escape route should lead to a place of safety, normally outside and away from the building

Compartmentation is necessary to contain a fire, and is particularly important in healthcare facilities. Compartmentation refers to the way the building is constructed to restrict the spread of fire and smoke by sub-dividing it into compartments separated from one another by walls and/or floors of fire-resistant construction.

There are two reasons for this:

1. To prevent rapid fire and smoke spread which could trap occupants in the building
2. To reduce the chance of the fire becoming large.

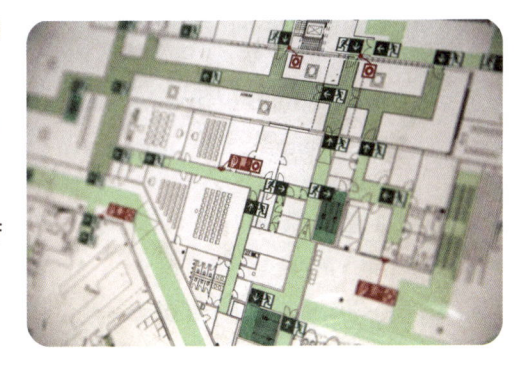

(HIQA 2016)

Compartmentation allows for a phased evacuation. Those who are at the greatest risk are evacuated directly to another part of the building through a fire door or doors into another compartment within the building. A phased evacuation strategy will naturally be the only realistic one in centres due to the difficulty in moving residents and potentially extended evacuation times.

Total evacuation is where all occupants of a building simultaneously evacuate upon hearing the alarm. This is appropriate for buildings where it may be expected, due to building size and/or capability of residents, that all people inside are able to (and will) evacuate quickly to a place of safety outside the building.

Personal Emergency Evacuation Plan (PEEP)

All staff must be aware of the purpose and function of the PEEP. For residents of designated centres who are not capable of responding to fire detection and alarm system activation and evacuating themselves without assistance, their needs and capabilities in the event of a fire should be assessed. This is usually done by way of a PEEP. The content should be agreed with the resident or representative as appropriate.

A PEEP should contain:

1. A current picture of the resident and pertinent information relating to him/her

2. Information on the capabilities of the resident in understanding the fire detection and alarm sounder

3. Information on the capabilities of the resident to evacuate and an outline of what staff need to do to help them as well as the method of evacuation (wheelchair/walking aids/other evacuation aids)

4. Information on any supervision requirements after the evacuation.

(HIQA 2016)

Emergency Procedures

Regardless of the location of a fire, once people are aware of it, they should be able to proceed safely along a recognisable escape route to a place of safety. Emergency procedure plans should always be guided by the principle that the time available for escape is greater than the time needed for escape.

- Under **Section 11 of the 2005 Act**, employers must prepare and revise adequate emergency plans and procedures and provide the necessary measures for firefighting and evacuating the workplace. Emergency procedures should be in place and practised to ensure safe evacuation in the event of a fire.

- **Sections 8, 9 and 10 of the 2005 Act** require that sufficient information, training and supervision is provided to ensure the safety of employees, taking into account any employees with specific needs, to ensure their protection against dangers that may affect them. Consideration for all employees and anyone connected with the workplace must form the basis of safety, health and welfare, with specific attention given to the provision of emergency access and egress.

- The **Workplace** chapter of the **Safety, Health and Welfare at Work (General Application) Regulations 2007** (the General Application Regulations) details fire safety requirements as follows: Regulation 11 – Doors and gates; Regulation 12 – Emergency routes and exits; Regulation 13 – Fire detection and firefighting; and Regulation 25 – Employees with disabilities.

- The **Safety Signs** chapter of the **General Application Regulations** contains requirements for fire-fighting equipment, emergency escape signs and fire-fighting signs.

- Fire detection, emergency lighting and emergency egress must also be addressed. Regulations require that 'emergency routes and exits requiring illumination are provided with emergency lighting of adequate intensity in case the lighting fails'.

- Two **National Standards Authority of Ireland** (NSAI) standards deal with **emergency lighting (I.S. 3217)** and **fire alarm installation (I.S. 3218)**.

(HSA website: 'Emergency Escape and Fire Fighting')

Emergency Escape and Fire-fighting Checklist

- Is an emergency plan in place for the workplace?
- Are regular fire drills conducted and monitored to put improvements in place?
- Are the extinguishers suitable for the purpose and of sufficient capacity?
- Are there sufficient extinguishers sited throughout the workplace?
- Are the right types of extinguisher located close to the fire hazards and can users gain access to them without exposing themselves to risk?
- Are signboards or a safety colour (or both) used to mark permanently the location and identification of fire-fighting equipment?
- Have the people likely to use the fire extinguishers been given adequate instruction and training?
- Is the use of fire-fighting equipment included in the emergency plan?

- Are all fire doors and escape routes and associated lighting and signs regularly checked?
- Is all fire-fighting equipment regularly checked?
- Is all other equipment provided to help means of escape arrangements in the building regularly checked?
- Are there instructions for relevant employees about testing of equipment?
- Are those who test and maintain the equipment properly trained to do so?

(HSA website: 'Emergency Escape and Fire Fighting')

The **Fire and Evacuation Drills for Management and Staff of the Fire Services Act 1981 (Section 4)** details actions that staff should be trained to take when a fire breaks out or when there is an alarm:

On discovering a fire:

- Operate the alarm system*
- Call the fire brigade
- Alert management and other staff
- Inform the public and direct them to the nearest available escape route
- Do not use the lift
- Attack the fire using the nearest suitable equipment (if safe to do so)
- Leave whenever danger threatens
- Close all doors as areas are vacated, checking that nobody is left behind

- Assemble at the designated assembly point
- Assist the fire brigade on arrival.

  * Where there is no alarm system, other means should be devised to signal to the occupants that a fire has occurred.

On hearing an alarm or other warning:

- Evacuate occupants using the nearest available escape route
- Do not use the lift
- Do not allow anybody to re-enter the premises for any reason
- Determine the location of the fire if possible
- Assemble at the designated assembly point
- Assist the fire brigade on arrival.

Case Study

Christopher and Laura are working in an 82-bed nursing home. On Thursday they are allocated to work in the 14-bed dementia unit together with a nurse. At around 10.30 a.m they hear the fire alarm go off; the procedure is that one of them goes to the panel to check where the fire is. Laura goes to check, and when she gets to the panel, other staff members are already there and inform her that the fire is located in room 12 of the dementia unit. Laura returns to the dementia unit with another staff member, and when they go down the hall, they notice smoke coming from under the door. They know that the resident in room 12 is in the day room with Christopher; however, since it is a dementia unit another resident could have wandered in. The nurse in charge alerts all care staff members that there is a fire.

Task

1. What action do the staff need to take?
2. Will the staff evacuate the entire nursing home or do a phased evacuation?
3. What are the complications in the scenario in terms of a total evacuation?

Quakers Hill Nursing Home Fire

The Quakers Hill Nursing Home fire was the most complex and intensive fire rescue operation undertaken by Fire and Rescue NSW, Australia, in many years. The actions of firefighters, ably assisted by nursing staff, police and ambulance, was instrumental in minimising deaths and injuries, but tragically 21 people lost their lives either during or following the fire.

At 4.53 a.m. on 18 November 2011, Fire and Rescue NSW (FRNSW) responded to an automatic fire alarm at the Quakers Hill Nursing Home in the west of Sydney. FRNSW sent 20 fire appliances and nearly 100 firefighters to the fire. Eighty-eight aged, sick and frail residents were physically rescued from the building. There were four staff members on duty who also assisted with the evacuation.

Two fires had been deliberately lit in separate wings. The first fire was minor and contained in an unoccupied room. The second fire was lit in an occupied room and spread throughout the wing. A nurse working in the home, Roger Dean, was later convicted of lighting the fires resulting in the murder of 11 residents. He was sentenced to life without parole.

In 2013, the NSW Government made installation of automatic fire sprinkler systems mandatory for all nursing homes.

Challenges for firefighters:

- Two separate fires caused initial confusion and delay, with both requiring separate intervention.

- Dense smoke descended to 50 cm above the floor in the ward, resulting in zero visibility.

- Some residents sought shelter under beds or behind furniture, making them difficult to locate.

- The alarm and building occupant warning system made communications difficult during the evacuation.

- Ceiling collapse created obstacles for rescuers.

- Mass rescue resulted in congestion at exits, particularly from moved beds. Many residents had to be carried from their beds at the exits.

- Fire/smoke doors in wards were opened as rescue took place, allowing dense smoke to enter the corridor and adjacent wards.

- Resources in the initial stages were limited and casualties could not receive immediate care.

- Lack of Triple Zero '000' call to confirm fire resulted in delay to escalated response.

Lessons for care facilities:

- Upon activation of fire alarm, staff should immediately check the source of the alarm to confirm the presence of smoke or fire.

- If fire is confirmed, it is vital that at least one person calls Triple Zero '000' so FRNSW can immediately respond with more resources.

- Staff must immediately begin staged evacuation, starting with those at greatest risk of harm.

- Staff must ensure fire/smoke doors remain closed to reduce fire and smoke spread.

- Mobile residents should be gathered in a safe area, then escorted to the assembly area if required by the nature of the emergency.

- Non-ambulant residents should be moved in accordance with the emergency plan. In extreme situations, residents may need to be carried or dragged to safety.

- During evacuation, passageways must be kept as clear as is reasonably practicable.

- Fire exits and other doors must be kept clear of obstructions at all times.

- Staff must give clear, concise instructions to residents during the evacuation, including visual gestures when background alarms make verbal communications impossible.

- The emergency plan must consider the evacuation of non-ambulant patients, such as those connected to medical equipment.

- Regular training and evacuation drills should be undertaken by all staff, including practising urgent removal of non-ambulant residents.

(Quoted, with permission, from Fire and Rescue NSW, Australia, https://www.fire.nsw.gov.au/page.php?id=9134)

A short news report on this fire can be viewed on YouTube: 'Quakers Hill nursing home fire' (Channel 10 (3:47)).

chapter 7
INFECTION PREVENTION AND CONTROL

> **IN THIS CHAPTER YOU WILL LEARN ABOUT:**
>
> + A range of issues related to infection control, including:
>   - conditions for the growth and development of micro-organisms
>   - routes of infection
>   - symptoms
>   - ill health
>   - preventive measures
>   - emergency procedures for suspected contamination

Microbiology

Microbiology is the study of tiny living things called micro-organisms. Micro-organisms include bacteria, viruses and fungi and are found everywhere: on people and animals, and in water, soil, food and air. Most micro-organisms are not harmful and live in or on our bodies without causing us any harm. Many play a vital role in digestion and in protecting us against invasion of other harmful micro-organisms.

Uses of micro-organisms include:

+ Moulds in the manufacture of antibiotics
+ Bacteria in the manufacture of cheese and yoghurts

- Viruses in medical research
- Yeast in the manufacture of beer.

Microbiological hazards, like all other workplace hazards, must be risk assessed to identify the hazard and assess the associated risk. Adequate control measures must then be implemented to eliminate the risk or reduce the risk to workers.

Pathogens

Pathogens are bacteria, viruses or micro-organisms that can cause disease when they enter the body. These may include minor infections that stay in one part of the body (localised) or infections that spread throughout the body (systemic), such as flu. Some infections are easily treated, but others can cause serious problems. Pathogens can be present on the body without invading tissue or causing infection. This is known as colonisation. Colonisation has no effect on the individual concerned, but it provides a source from which the pathogen can be easily transferred to another person and subsequently cause infection.

Opportunistic pathogens cause infection if they gain access to the human body, but the severity of the illness is dependent on the vulnerability of the host, e.g. elderly, very young or immune-compromised people suffer more severely. MRSA may be described as an opportunistic pathogen as those at greatest risk are older people, very young people, those with reduced immunity to infection (HIV clients or anti-cancer therapy clients), those who have had a recent acute illness and long-term residents of healthcare facilities.

Types of Micro-organism

Micro-organisms include bacteria, viruses, fungi and parasites.

Bacteria are tiny living things that cannot be seen by the naked eye as they are too small; they can only be viewed under a microscope. In the healthcare environment, microbiological hazards must be reduced to a safe level to prevent the spread of infection and disease. Common healthcare-associated bacterial infections are MRSA, *Clostridium difficile* (*C.diff*), legionella (Legionnaires' disease), vancomycin-resistant Enterococcus (VRE) and tuberculosis (TB). Bacterial hazards in a kitchen include *E. coli*, *Salmonella*, *Listeria* and *Campylobacter*.

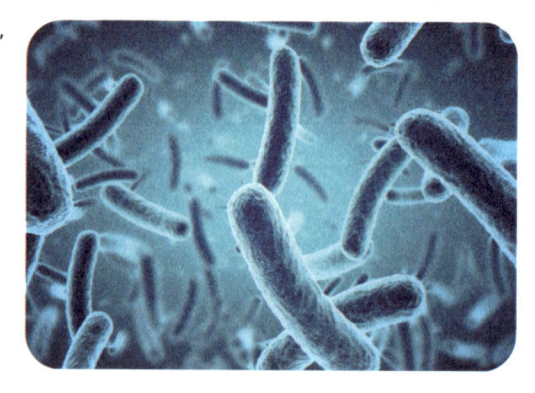

Viruses are even smaller than bacteria. They are also more difficult to kill. The main difference between a virus and a bacterium is the way they reproduce. Unlike bacteria, viruses cannot reproduce by themselves; they can only replicate themselves inside a living cell. They are dependent on the host cell for growth. Common healthcare-associated viruses include Norovirus (winter vomiting bug), Covid-19 (coronavirus), SARS, hepatitis B, hepatitis C and HIV.

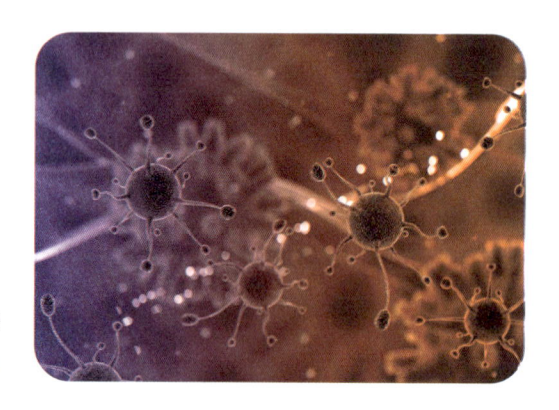

ADULT EDUCATION SERVICE BALBRIGGAN

2 4 NOV 2020

ADULT EDUCATION SERVICE BALBRIGGAN
SARSFIELD HOUSE, MILL STREET
BALBRIGGAN CO. DUBLIN K32KX82
TEL: 01-8417763

Fungi are another type of micro-organism. Some (e.g. mushrooms) can be seen with the naked eye; others can only be seen under a microscope. Infections caused by fungi can be superficial and affect body surfaces, e.g. skin, hair and nails; they include athlete's foot, thrush and ringworm.

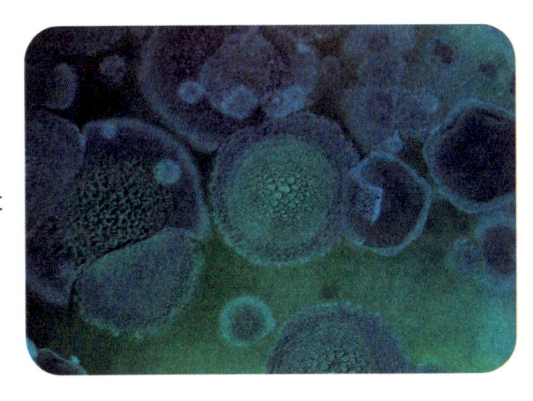

Some bacteria can develop highly resistant structures called **spores**. Spores are resistant to disinfectants and to high and low temperatures. They can remain viable for several years. They are a particularly challenging micro-biological hazard to manage, if environmental conditions allow the spores to germinate and the bacterial cell inside starts to multiply. Bacterial spores can survive in dust for long periods of time, e.g. *C. diff*. Environmental contamination from *C. diff* has been positively identified as the source of infection in reported outbreaks in a healthcare setting.

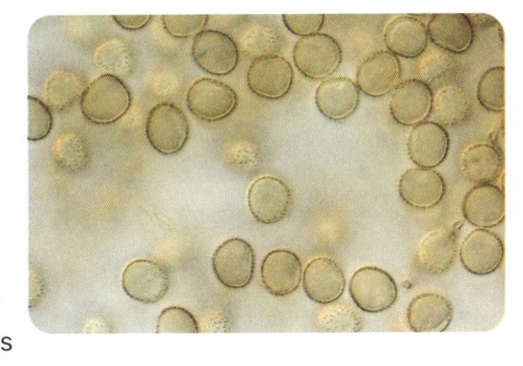

A **parasite** is an organism that lives on or in a host organism and gets its food from or at the expense of its host. There are three main types of parasite that can cause disease in humans: protozoa, helminths and ectoparasites.

Protozoan infections are responsible for diseases that affect many different types of organism, including plants, animals and some marine life. Deadly human diseases caused by a protozoan infection include African sleeping sickness, amoebic dysentery and malaria.

Helminths are worm-like parasites, for example tapeworms. Tapeworms are segmented flatworms that attach themselves to the insides of the intestines of animals such as cows, pigs and humans. They get food by eating the host's partly digested food, depriving the host of nutrients.

Ectoparasites broadly include blood-sucking arthropods such as mosquitoes (because they are dependent on a blood meal from a human host for their survival), but this term is used more narrowly to refer to ticks, fleas, lice and mites that attach or burrow into the skin and remain there for relatively long periods of time (weeks or months). Arthropods are important in causing diseases, but are even more important as vectors or transmitters of many different pathogens that in turn cause tremendous morbidity and mortality from the diseases they cause.

(CDCP website)

Growth and Development of Micro-organisms

To prevent the growth and multiplication of pathogenic bacteria we must first understand the requirements for bacterial growth. As with all other living creatures, bacteria need food and water for growth and multiplication. Most will not survive for long on clean, dry surfaces but will readily multiply on poorly cleaned equipment, in dirty water, and even in certain solutions of disinfectant.

Under the right conditions, bacteria split in two approximately every twenty minutes in a process known as binary fission. This is known as an asexual form of reproduction as it does not involve a male and female. Each cell produces two identical cells, which will in turn split in two if conditions remain favourable.

The requirements for bacterial growth are:

- **Time:** In a ten-hour period one single cell will become one billion bacterial cells if the conditions are right.
- **Warmth:** For each species of bacteria there is a specific temperature range within which growth takes place. Some grow well at room temperature or even body temperature (37°C).
- **Oxygen:** Some bacteria are aerobic (need oxygen to survive) and some can only survive in the absence of oxygen (anaerobic).
- **Food:** Like all living things, bacteria require food to thrive and grow.
- **Moisture:** Bacteria require moist conditions in order to multiply. Bacteria will not multiply on dry surfaces or equipment.

Spread of Micro-organisms

In the healthcare environment micro-organisms can be spread either directly or indirectly.

Direct contact is when micro-organisms are transferred from one person to another by direct contact between body surfaces, e.g. through blood or other bodily fluid or through sexual contact. Puncture wounds from sharps, including needles, syringes and razor blades, that have been contaminated by blood from infected clients can lead to viral infections such as hepatitis B and hepatitis C, which cause inflammation of the liver. HIV can also be contracted through a needle-stick injury from an infected client.

Indirect contact involves the transfer of a micro-organism by means of a vehicle, i.e. a contaminated object or piece of equipment. Micro-organisms can be indirectly transferred by the following vehicles:

- **Hands:** The spread of pathogenic bacteria in this way can easily be prevented by carrying out the correct level of hand hygiene.

- **Equipment and inanimate objects:** Micro-organisms can be carried on phones, door handles, wheels of equipment, cleaning equipment, etc.

- **Airborne particles:** Pathogenic micro-organisms can be carried on airborne particles such as respiratory droplets water and dust. Practising good cough and sneezing etiquette can contribute to the containment of respiratory droplets.

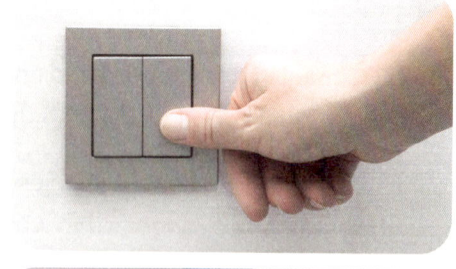

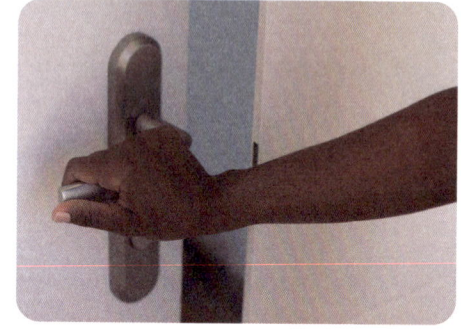

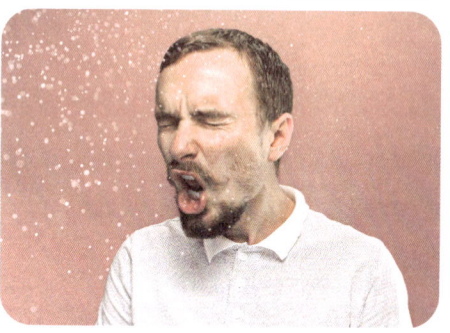

- **Vectors (an organism, typically a biting insect or tick):** Animals or insects can carry harmful bacteria on their feet, coat, fur or bodies and are often involved in transmission to humans.

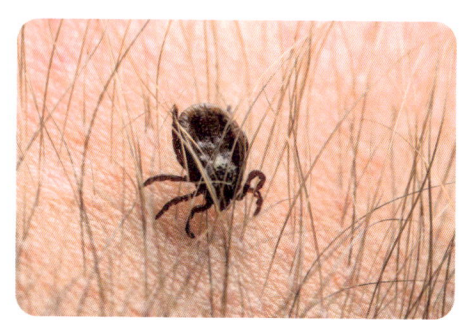

- **Food and water:** Some foods, either in a ready-to-eat or raw state, can harbour pathogenic bacteria and when consumed by vulnerable clients can cause food poisoning. Common food poisoning bacteria are *Salmonella*, *E. coli*, and *Listeria*. Food workers suffering from gastrointestinal upset should not attend work as harmful bacteria can be transmitted via the hands to clients and co-workers. Micro-organisms can also be transmitted through contaminated water, e.g. *Cryptosporidium*.

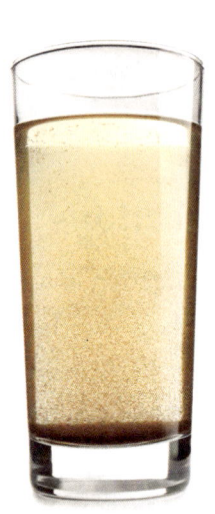

> Hand hygiene following the delivery of direct contact and indirect contact care is essential in preventing the spread of infection.

Transient and Resident Micro-organisms

Transient micro-organisms are found on the skin surface and live for only a short period of time. They can be easily passed from one person to another and cause infection unless they are removed. These types of organisms can be carried on the hands of healthcare workers and equipment and are commonly associated with healthcare-associated infections (HCAIs).

Correct hand hygiene can easily remove them and reduce/remove the risk of contamination.

Resident micro-organisms live much deeper in the skin or in the nose and for the most part are harmless. They are part of our immune system, protect us from infection and are not normally associated with HCAIs. However, vulnerable clients who may be immuno-compromised can be susceptible to infection from this type of micro-organism.

Infections

An infection is an invasion of harmful micro-organisms into the body, resulting in illness or disease. The infection can be localised or systemic. Transmission of micro-organisms can be through the faecal-oral route, via vehicles (e.g. equipment), droplets, non-human carriers, blood and bodily fluids and through the air. Micro-organisms can enter the body and from here they will grow and multiply, with signs and symptoms of infection becoming apparent. For infection to occur a series of events must happen. This series of events is known as the **chain of infection**. There are six links in the chain of infection and each link must connect for an infection to occur.

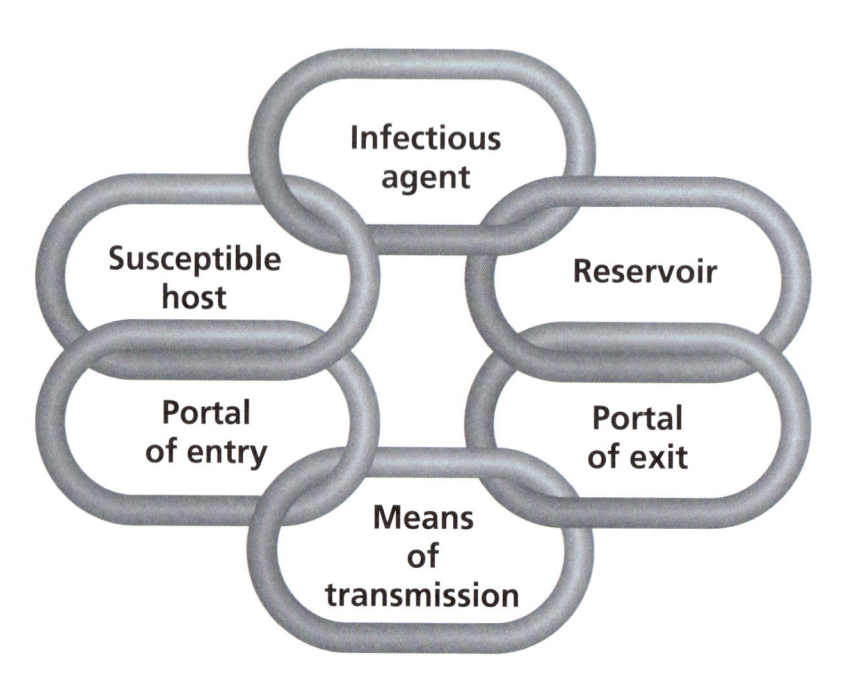

Chain of Infection

In the healthcare setting our aim is to prevent infection and reduce the risk to clients, staff and the public by breaking the chain of infection. To break the chain of infection, healthcare workers must understand each link and how they connect to cause infection in a host. An infectious agent can be a bacterium, virus, fungus or parasite. If all the links in the chain of infection are present, any micro-organism can cause an infection. As we know already, micro-organisms are everywhere in the environment and are also carried by humans and animals.

Elements in the chain of infection are:

+ **Reservoir:** Where the infectious agent lives and reproduces, e.g. people, water, food, animals and insects.

+ **Portal of exit:** The means by which the infectious agent leaves the host. This can be through the respiratory tract (coughing, sneezing, talking), non-intact skin (wounds that have an exudate, including pressure sores), gastrointestinal tract (vomiting and diarrhoea) and mucus membranes (eyes, nose and mouth).

+ **Mode of transmission:** The way in which the micro-organism travels from the reservoir to the host. This can be direct or indirect.

+ **Portal of entry:** Where the infectious agents enter the host, e.g. non-intact skin, the respiratory tract or through exposure to a contaminated sharp object through a needle-stick injury.

+ **Susceptible host:** The person who becomes infected by the infectious agent. Individuals who have never been exposed to the micro-organism can become ill because they do not have antibodies to protect them. This protection can be achieved through immunisation or through previous infection.

The chain of infection can be broken in the following ways:

- Correct hand-washing technique
- Segregation of healthcare
- Segregation of healthcare linen
- Control of dust
- Keeping equipment clean
- Environmental cleaning
- Use of appropriate PPE
- Pest control.

Healthcare-Associated Infections (HCAIs)

HCAIs are infections that clients acquire during the course of receiving healthcare treatment for other conditions (CDCP website). This infection would not have been present or incubating at the time of admission. If a client gets sick within 48 hours of having been admitted to the healthcare facility, they are likely to have brought the infection with them.

Pre-disposing factors that make one client more susceptible to a HCAI than others include:

- Clients with large wounds, following surgery, a burns injury or a serious accident, e.g. a road traffic accident (RTA)
- Clients who are on a drip (intravenous line) or other medical devices for a long time, e.g. infusion pump, enteral feeding, ventilation, dialysis

- Clients with a weakened immune system, such as clients that are being treated/have recently been treated for leukaemia or cancer or have been the recipient of an organ transplant

- Clients at either extreme of age, i.e. the very young or very old, both groups being more vulnerable than other age groups

- The presence of antibiotic-resistant strains of bacteria, which are more likely to prevail in a hospital environment and also spread from person to person, due to clients being more likely to receive antibiotics for infection or as a prophylaxis (preventative measure) against infection prior to surgery.

Common HCAIs include MRSA, *C.diff* infection, Norovirus, Legionnaires' disease, blood-borne viruses, tuberculosis and Covid-19 (coronavirus).

MRSA

Methicillin-resistant *Staphylococcus aureus* (MRSA) is a strand of *S. aureus* that has developed resistance to many antibiotics commonly used to treat *Staphylococcus* infections, and as a result can be difficult to treat. *S. aureus* colonises the nose and skin of healthy people, and the groin and perineum. About 20 per cent of people can have the organism most of the time and a further 60 per cent carry it intermittently. It can cause serious infection if it enters damaged skin or surgical wounds.

MRSA can be carried on the hands of healthcare workers and spread through direct contact. Clothing and equipment may also be involved in the transmission, but the environment is not considered to play an important role in transmission in most settings.

Individuals with a weakened immune system or open wounds are more susceptible to MRSA than healthier members of the population.

Hand washing is acknowledged as being the single most important factor in the fight to prevent MRSA infections. Where possible, affected clients should be nursed in a single room and staff must ensure that correct hand hygiene techniques are utilised before and after contact with an MRSA client and their environment. Where it is not possible to place all MRSA colonised/infected clients in a single room, a risk assessment must be conducted to inform and provide staff with the evidence to prioritise and provide suitable accommodation to prevent potential adverse outcomes for all clients, staff and visitors.

Clostridium Difficile

C.diff is a common inhabitant of the human gut, but exposure to antibiotics can allow it to multiply and disturb the balance of flora in the gut. The route of transmission is direct and indirect contact with faeces. The client infected with *C.diff* will present with bloody diarrhoea; some cases are fatal. *C.diff* spores are resistant to many cleaning agents and can survive in the environment for prolonged periods of time. Correct and frequent hand hygiene is recommended when dealing with *C.diff* clients. Alcohol gels are not effective against *C.diff* spores.

Norovirus

Norovirus is transmitted by hands contaminated through the faecal-oral route, directly from person to person or through contaminated food or water. It can also be transmitted through contaminated surfaces, e.g. door handles.

Using the correct hand-washing technique for at least 20 seconds has been proven to be an effective method of preventing the spread of Norovirus. Sanitising alcohol gels can also be used, provided that hands are visibly clean.

Legionnaires' Disease

According to the HSE, about ten cases of Legionnaires' disease are reported each year. It is most common in people over 50 years of age with compromised immune systems. It occurs when the bacterium *Legionella* gets access to a water system, shower heads or water fountains and can multiply if conditions are right. Chlorination does not kill these bacteria. It can be contracted by inhaling droplets or spray from water systems that have been contaminated, for example using a shower that has not been used for some time and in which stagnant water has been at optimum temperatures for bacterial growth. Legionnaires' disease starts with flu-like symptoms, fever, aches and pains, followed by a dry cough and breathing difficulties and can progress to severe pneumonia.

Elimination of the risk of contracting Legionnaires' disease can be achieved by regular cleaning and maintenance of water distribution systems. Particular attention in a healthcare facility should be given to areas of the buildings that are infrequently used.

Blood-borne Viruses

Blood-borne pathogens are infectious micro-organisms in human blood that can cause disease in humans. They include hepatitis B, hepatitis C and human immunodeficiency virus (HIV).

Hepatitis B and Hepatitis C

Hepatitis B is a potentially life-threatening liver infection caused by the hepatitis B virus (HBV). It can cause chronic liver disease and place people at a high risk of death from cirrhosis of the liver and liver cancer. Exposure to hepatitis B is possible through:

- Blood transfusions
- Direct contact with blood in a healthcare setting

- Sexual contact with an infected person
- Tattoos or acupuncture using unclean instruments or needles
- Shared needles during drug use
- Shared personal items such as toothbrushes, razors or nail clippers.

Many people may not know they are carrying the virus; however, they can still spread it. Healthcare workers must assess all clients on an individual basis to ensure appropriate client management and reducing risk to staff and clients. Early symptoms may include loss of appetite, tiredness, low-grade fever, muscle and joint pain, nausea and vomiting, and yellow skin and dark urine.

All staff in healthcare should be vaccinated against hepatitis B.

All control measures should be in place when caring for a client infected with the HBV. All bloodstained items and PPE from infected clients must be disposed of as healthcare risk waste. Appropriate use of PPE and hand hygiene techniques must be exercised by staff as per best practice and training.

Hepatitis C is caused by the hepatitis C virus (HCV). Its method of transmission is the same as HBV. Currently there is no vaccine for active immunisation against HCV. Control measures are the same as those for HBV.

Human Immunodeficiency Virus (HIV)

HIV is acquired through sexual contact, inoculation of blood or body fluids through the skin by contaminated needles or other sharp items, and exposure of mucus membranes. The virus is present in blood, semen, vaginal secretions, cerebrospinal fluid, amniotic fluid and synovial fluid. Healthcare workers are at risk through needle-stick injuries or contamination from blood or body fluids. Control measures must be in place as with all blood-borne viruses.

Tuberculosis

This is a contagious airborne infectious disease that generally affects the lungs through inhalation and is predominantly spread through coughing, sneezing, spitting or talking that expels air and dispersing droplets that contain *Mycobacterium tuberculosis* (*M.tb*).

Control measures against the spread of TB include:

- Vaccination

- Engineering controls (positive/negative atmospheric pressure, direct negative airflow coming from the corridor and exhausted to the exterior of the building). New or refurbished healthcare settings should contain isolation rooms for clients with active TB. This prevents the spread of TB nuclei to the remainder of the building.

- Administrative controls: staff training at induction to include familiarisation with the symptoms of TB and at regular intervals thereafter. Staff required to come into direct contact with infectious clients by entering isolation rooms must be offered additional protection. This is dictated by local policy but will include the use of FFP1, FFP2 and FFP3 respirators. Clients leaving isolation, e.g. to go for a diagnostic investigation, will also be required to wear the respirators.

- PPE, appropriate application and disposal as healthcare risk waste.

Covid-19 (Coronavirus)

Coronavirus disease (Covid-19) is a new infectious disease caused by coronavirus. The Covid-19 virus spreads primarily through droplets of saliva or discharge from the nose when an infected person coughs or sneezes. It can also be transmitted by touching surfaces that someone who has the virus has coughed or sneezed on. Currently (as of September 2020), there are no specific vaccines or treatments for Covid-19, but there are many ongoing clinical trials evaluating potential treatments.

Typical symptoms of coronavirus include fever and a cough that may progress to a severe pneumonia causing shortness of breath and breathing difficulties. Current estimates suggest that the time between exposure to the virus and developing symptoms (the incubation period) is from five to six days but can range from one to 14 days. Staff members who test positive for Covid-19 may return to work 14 days after symptom onset (or date of diagnosis if no symptoms) provided they have had no fever during the previous five days.

Most people infected with the Covid-19 virus will experience mild to moderate respiratory illness and recover without requiring special treatment. However, older people and those with underlying medical problems like cardiovascular disease, diabetes, chronic respiratory disease and cancer are more likely to develop a serious illness.

(WHO website)

To prevent infection and to slow the transmission of Covid-19, healthcare workers must:

- Attend training in standard precautions, hand hygiene, respiratory hygiene and cough etiquette and in transmission-based precautions (contact, droplet and airborne) including the appropriate use of PPE

- Wash their hands regularly with soap and water or clean them with alcohol-based hand rub

- Maintain at least one-metre distance between themselves and people coughing or sneezing

- Encourage residents to maintain a one- to two-metre distance from other residents and staff. They should also be advised to avoid touching other people (touching hands, hugging, kissing).

- Cover their mouth and nose when coughing or sneezing.

(HSPC website)

> **Activity**
>
> Pick a healthcare-related illness.
>
> - Outline the causes of the illness.
> - Discuss its symptoms.
> - Describe how the illness could have an impact on a healthcare worker.
> - How could a healthcare worker prevent the illness?

Preventive Measures and Emergency Procedures for Suspected Contamination

Standard Precautions

Standard precautions are a set of general infection control guidelines that all healthcare staff must follow during delivery of care to clients. These precautions should always be used during care delivery. Standard precaution guidelines provide the foundation for infection prevention and control practices.

The aim of the guidelines is to ensure that the chain of infection is not complete and to prevent the transmission of common infectious agents. Standard precautions assume that infectious agents could be present in the client's blood, body fluids, secretions, excretions, non-intact skin and mucous membranes.

Standard precautions include:

- Hand washing
- Waste management and decontamination issues
- Management of linen
- Respiratory hygiene and cough etiquette
- Appropriate use of PPE.

Transmission-based Precautions

When transmissible infectious agents require additional controls, transmission-based precautions must be used in addition to standard precautions. Organisms/infectious agents that require additional controls (in conjunction with standard precautions) to reduce the risk of adverse outcomes for clients, staff and the public are:

- MRSA
- *Clostridium difficile*
- Tuberculosis
- Norovirus
- H1N1 (flu virus/pandemic)
- *Salmonella*
- Chicken pox
- Measles.

Transmission-based precautions include contact precautions, airborne precautions and droplet precautions.

Contact Precautions

These precautions should be applied in addition to standard precautions to prevent transmission of highly transmissible organisms that are transmitted from person to person via the contact routes, e.g. MRSA.

Contact precautions deal with both direct and indirect contact (via a vehicle) and contact through vectors. The following controls must be put in place when using contact precautions:

- Isolation room if available
- If unavailable, contact the infection prevention and control nurse (IPCN) or the clinical nurse manager in charge
- PPE: gloves and gown for all interactions
- Care of client and client equipment
- Decontamination of equipment and the environment
- Hand hygiene.

Airborne Precautions

Airborne precautions should be used in addition to standard precautions to prevent transmission of highly transmissible organisms that are transmitted via the air from one person to another, e.g. tuberculosis, measles and chicken pox.

(HPSC 2007)

Airborne precautions include:

- Airborne infection isolation room with adequate air exchanges per hour

- Use of appropriate face masks as per local policy
- Correct fitting of appropriate mask/respirator prior to entry into the client's room
- Removal of mask only after leaving the client's room
- Wearing of the appropriate mask by client if they have to leave their room
- Staff training.

Droplet Precautions

These precautions should be applied, in addition to standard precautions, to prevent the transmission of highly transmissible organisms that are transmitted via respiratory secretions from one person to another, e.g. influenza.

(HSE 2020)

Droplet precautions aim to prevent the transmission of pathogens spread through close respiratory or mucous membrane secretions.

Controls include:

- Single room preferred
- If not possible, spatial separation of more than one metre is required; drawing the curtain between client beds is especially important for clients in multi-bed rooms
- PPE: surgical mask if within one metre of the client
- Client to wear face mask before leaving their isolation room.

Healthcare Linen

Linen or laundry that has been used in a healthcare environment must be treated as a potential infection risk and needs to be segregated appropriately. All linen falls into one of three groups:

- Clean/unused linen
- Dirty/used linen
- Foul/infected linen.

Handling/Storage of Clean Linen

- Clean linen is any linen that has not been used since it was last laundered.
- All clean linen must be stored off the floor in a clean, closed cupboard and must be segregated from dirty/used linen.
- Clean linen must not be stored in the sluice or bathroom.
- Linen cupboard doors must be kept closed to prevent airborne contamination.
- Clean/unused linen should be delivered to wards in clean containers; these containers should not then be used to collect used linen.
- If taken into an isolation room and not used, linen must be laundered before use.

Handling/Storage of Dirty Linen

- All dirty linen must be handled with care, to minimise transmission of micro-organisms via dust and skin scales.
- Plastic aprons should be worn when there is the potential for contamination of clothing, i.e. when changing beds.

- All dirty linen must be placed carefully and directly into the appropriate laundry bag (white bag) on removal from the bed or client.

- Bring the laundry skip to the bedside and place the dirty linen into the appropriate bag.

- Hands must be washed immediately following the handling of any dirty or contaminated linen.

- To avoid spillage of dirty linen, linen bags must never be more than two-thirds full.

- Bags must be secured appropriately for transporting to the laundry.

- Vehicles or trolleys used to transport dirty or contaminated linen must be easy to clean and must never be used to transport clean linen.

Handling Foul/Infected Linen

- Infected linen includes bed linen which is soiled with blood or any other body fluid, or linen used by a client with a known infection (soiled or not).

- All infected linen must be handled with care, to minimise transmission of micro-organisms via dust and skin scales.

- Plastic aprons and gloves must be worn when handling infected linen.

- All infected bed linen must be placed into a water-soluble/alginate stitch bag (orange/colourless).

- The water soluble/alginate stitch bag is then put into a red linen bag for transportation.

- Linen bags must never be more than two-thirds full.

CHAPTER 07: INFECTION PREVENTION AND CONTROL

- The water soluble/alginate stitch bag must be placed directly into the washing machine and not opened before washing.
- Hands must be washed immediately after handling any dirty or contaminated linen.

Task 1

Áine is a resident in a 32-bed nursing home. She contracted MRSA while in hospital and is recuperating in the nursing home.

Searlait has been a care assistant in this nursing home for the past two years. She has completed Care Skills and Care of the Older Person QQI modules, but not Infection Prevention and Control.

Today it is Searlait's duty to wash Áine and get her ready for the day. This also involves changing the linen on Áine's bed.

Searlait enters Áine's room without wearing any gloves or PPE. She strips the bed, walks up the corridor with the used linen and throws them into the laundry basket. Then she grabs a new clean set of sheets for the bed and returns to the room to remake the bed.

1. What type of PPE should Searlait have when worn entering the room?
2. What category does Áines linen fall into?
3. How should Searlait handle the infected linen?
4. How should the linen be transported to the laundry room?
5. What should Searlait do before handling clean linen?

chapter 8
SAFETY EQUIPMENT

IN THIS CHAPTER YOU WILL LEARN ABOUT:

- How personal protective equipment (PPE) is used in the workplace
- The typical contents of a first aid kit and their appropriate use
- The importance of signage
- Signs and their meaning

Personal Protective Equipment (PPE)

The **Safety, Health and Welfare at Work (General Application) Regulations 2007 (Part 2, Chapter 3)** covers use of PPE work. PPE is any device or appliance designed to be worn or held by an individual for protection against one or more health and safety hazard. Respiratory protective equipment (RPE) is a type of PPE that is used to protect the wearer against inhalation of hazardous substances in the workplace air.

Where there is a risk to the safety, health and welfare of employees, the employer has a duty to avoid or limit such risk by methods of prevention or implementation of control systems of work. PPE should only be provided where the risks cannot be avoided or limited by other means.

The employer must assess the hazards in the workplace to identify the correct type of PPE to be provided and to ensure that it is appropriate to the risk. Care must be exercised in selecting PPE, as certain types give reasonably high levels of protection while others, which may appear almost the same, give relatively low levels of protection.

The **European Union (Personal Protective Equipment) Regulations 2018** provide that PPE may not be placed on the market or brought into service unless it complies with basic health and safety requirements and bears the CE mark.

Provision of PPE in the Workplace

Section 8 of the Safety, Health and Welfare at Work Act 2005 places a duty on employers to supply PPE where risks cannot be eliminated or adequately controlled.

- Employers cannot pass on to employees any financial costs associated with duties relating to safety, health and welfare at work. An employer may not ask for money to be paid to them by an employee for the provision of PPE, whether returnable (e.g. a deposit) or otherwise.
- Employers may charge a worker for PPE if the worker is truly self-employed.
- Where an employee wishes to upgrade to a more expensive item of PPE (e.g. the employee wants a more fashionable brand), the employer and employee may enter into an agreement whereby the employee makes up the difference between the cost of the original item of PPE and that of the more expensive item, assuming they both give the same level of protection.

Training in the Use of PPE

- Where PPE is provided, employees must be informed of the risks against which they are being protected by the PPE.
- Employees must also be provided with suitable information, instruction and training (including training in the use, care

or maintenance of PPE) to enable them to make proper and effective use of any PPE provided for their protection.

- PPE users must be trained as regards the wearing, proper use and any limitations of PPE.

- Managers and supervisors should also be aware of the reasons for providing PPE, its proper use and the level of protection afforded.

- Training, both theoretical and practical, should also be given to those involved in the selection, maintenance, repair and testing of PPE.

- The level of training provided will vary with the level of risk involved and the complexity and use of the equipment. For instance, the use of respirator equipment will require a comprehensive degree of training with regular refresher courses, whereas the training for using protective gloves for dealing with hazardous substances may require demonstration only. The frequency of the refresher courses required in the case of PPE for high-risk situations will depend on the nature of the equipment, how frequently it is used and the needs of the employees using it.

PPE Users

There is a duty on employees, having regard to their training and instructions, to make correct use of PPE. Employees should:

- Use PPE properly whenever it is required to be used

- Report any defects in or damage to the PPE immediately

- Participate in any PPE training or instruction provided

- Inform their employer of any medical conditions they have that might be affected by the use of the PPE provided to them.

When to Use PPE

+ The fundamental principle is that PPE should only be used as a last resort.

+ The safety and health of employees must be first safeguarded by measures to eliminate workplace risks at source, through technical or organisational means (e.g. by substituting hazardous chemicals) or by providing protection on a collective basis (e.g. providing training in client moving and handling).

+ Collective protective measures covering numbers of employees in a workplace must have priority over protective measures applying to individual employees.

+ If these measures are not sufficient, only then should PPE be used to protect against the hazards that are unavoidable.

PPE has its limitations because:

+ PPE protects the wearer only

+ It is ineffective if not working or fitted properly

+ Theoretical levels of protection are seldom reached in practice

+ The use of PPE always restricts the wearer to some degree

+ The psychological effect of PPE may be such that the individual wearing the PPE feels more protected than he or she actually is

+ If PPE is not working or not fitted properly, the person wearing it is exposed to the risk as this is the only (or last) protection they have against the particular hazard.

PPE Testing, Inspection and Storage

+ PPE must be thoroughly examined regularly by competent staff according to the manufacturer's instructions. As a general rule, simple maintenance may be carried out by the user, provided that he or she has been adequately instructed and trained (e.g. cleaning goggles lenses or replacing helmet straps).

+ The examination, maintenance and repair of PPE used in high-risk situations should be carried out by properly trained staff or the manufacturer or supplier (or both). Those involved should have the necessary tools and materials to carry out proper repairs.

+ PPE must be stored according to the manufacturer's instructions. This is extremely important as leaving PPE lying around increases the risk of parts deteriorating by exposure to dirt, oil, UV rays, sunlight, etc.

(HSA website: 'PPE – FAQs')

Types of PPE for Healthcare Workers

Healthcare workers should wear protective clothing when there is a risk of contact with blood, body fluids, secretions and excretions (with the exception of sweat). They should select the appropriate PPE (gloves, apron/gown, eye, nose and mouth protection) based on a risk assessment of the task to be carried out. Protective clothing can create a false sense of security and even increase the risk of cross-infection if used incorrectly, e.g. failure to carry out hand hygiene following the removal of gloves.

1. **Gloves** reduce the risk of contamination but do not eliminate it, so gloves are not a substitute for performing hand hygiene. Gloves should be worn for:

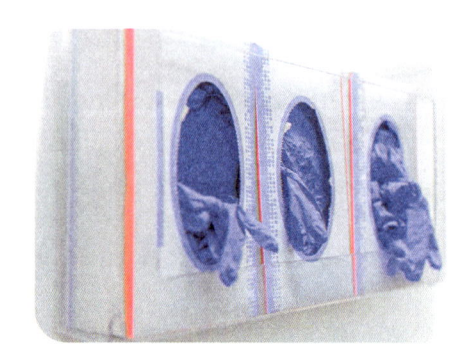

- All activities that have been assessed as carrying a risk of exposure to blood, body fluids, secretions (except sweat) and excretions

- Direct contact with sterile sites, non-intact skin or mucous membranes

- Handling sharp or contaminated instruments and equipment

- Invasive procedures.

2. **Disposable plastic aprons** should be worn when there is a risk that clothing or uniform may become contaminated with blood, body fluids, secretions (except sweat) or excretions. Aprons are single use and should be discarded after the procedure or episode of care, and hand hygiene carried out.

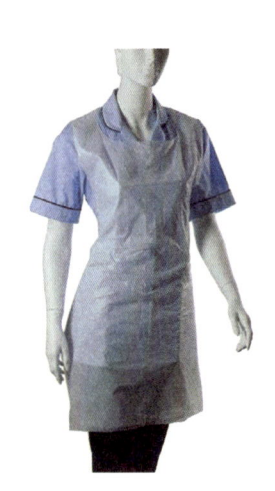

3. **Facial protection** – face /mouth/ eye protection. A fluid-repellent mask and protective eyewear or a face shield to protect the mucous membranes of the eyes, nose and mouth should be worn during any procedure or client care activity where there is a risk of blood and/or body fluids splashing onto the face, e.g. irrigation of a wound or suctioning.

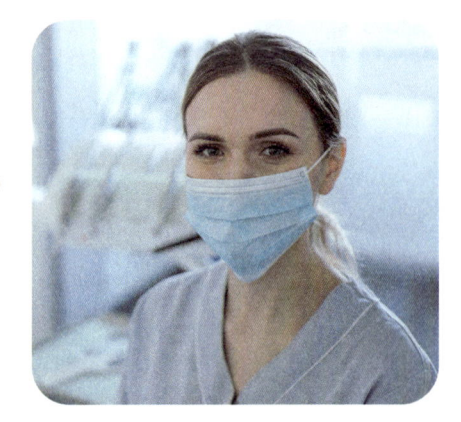

4. **Footwear** Healthcare workers should wear enclosed footwear that can protect them from injuries with sharp objects if sharps are accidentally dropped.

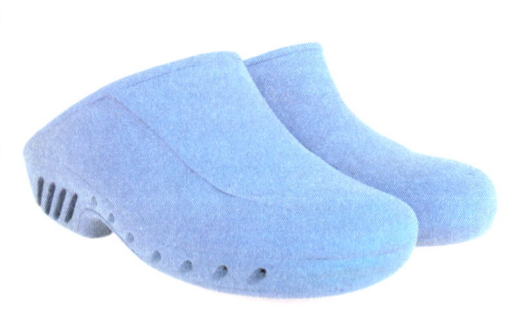

Donning and Removing PPE

The type of PPE used will vary based on the risk of exposure anticipated, and not all items of PPE will be required at the same time. Hand hygiene should be performed before and after putting on PPE.

The order for **putting on** PPE is:

1. Apron or gown
2. Fluid-repellent face mask
3. Eye protection
4. Gloves.

When the procedure is complete, **remove** PPE in the following order:

1. Remove gloves
2. Remove apron/gown
3. Decontaminate hands
4. Remove eyewear
5. Remove mask without touching the front of the mask

CHAPTER 08: SAFETY EQUIPMENT

6. Decontaminate hands
7. Dispose of PPE carefully and in the correct bins/receptacle.

> **Task**
>
> Matthew is a care assistant and he is working in a nursing home where there is a case of the mumps. Matthew is concerned as his wife is eight months pregnant.
>
> + What precautions can Matthew take so that he does not contract mumps?
> + What PPE should Matthew use if in contact with the resident who has mumps?

First Aid Kit

First aid is the provision of immediate care to a victim with an injury or illness, usually performed by a lay person, and performed within a limited skill range. First aid is normally performed until the injury or illness is satisfactorily dealt with (such as in the case of small cuts, minor bruises and blisters) or until the next level of care, such as a paramedic or doctor, arrives.

Guiding principles

The key guiding principles and purpose of first aid are the three Ps. These three points govern all the actions undertaken by a first aider.

+ **P**revent further injury
+ **P**reserve life
+ **P**romote recovery

A standard first aid kit comes in a green polypropylene case and contains first aid treatments for all minor cuts and injuries and is ideal for workplaces, schools and colleges.

The number of first aid kits needed for the workplace should be based on the following factors:

- The size of the premises
- The types of activity being carried out
- Frequency of accidents arising
- Existence of special hazards
- Distance from nearest appropriate medical facility.

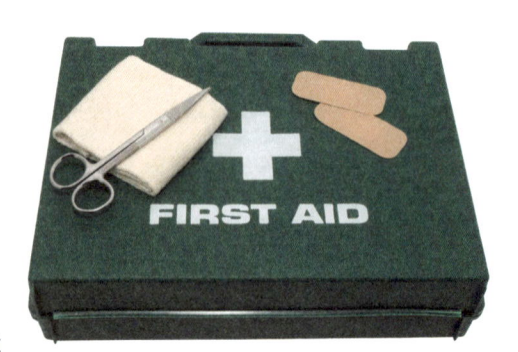

First Aid Kit Contents

	1–10 Persons	11–25 Persons	26–50 Persons	Travel Kit
Assorted adhesive plasters	20	20	40	20
Triangular bandages	2	6	6	2
No. 8 dressing	2	2	4	1
No. 9 dressing	2	6	8	1
No. 3 dressing (extra large)	2	3	4	1
Eye pad dressing	2	2	4	2
Disinfectant cleansing wipes	10	20	40	10
Crepe bandage (7 cm)	1	2	3	1
Safety pins	6	6	6	6
Pocket face mask	1	1	1	1

	1–10 Persons	11–25 Persons	26–50 Persons	Travel Kit
Paramedic shears	1	1	1	1
Gloves (pairs)	5	10	10	3

Kits with eye wash and burns dressings include:

Sterile water	250 ml	250 ml	250 ml	2 x 20 ml
Small burns dressing (10 x 10 cm)	1	1	1	1
Large burns dressing (10 x 40 cm)	1	1	1	1

(Guide to the Safety, Health and Welfare at Work [General Application] Regulations 2007, Chapter 2 of Part 7: First Aid)

First aid does not cover the administration of drugs or medications, and painkillers/headache tablets should not be kept in the workplace first aid kit. In certain circumstances, first aiders can assist in the administration of aspirin if available for suspected cardiac chest pain.

First Aid Records and Documentation

The names of occupational first aiders must be recorded in the safety statement along with the location of the first aid rooms, equipment and facilities.

Written records of the dates of all first aid training, including refresher training, should be kept at the workplace and be made available on request to the Health and Safety Inspector.

Records of all cases treated by the first aider should be kept in a suitable, secure place, respecting their confidential nature, and be made available on request to the health and safety inspector.

Automated External Defibrillator (AED)

A defibrillator is a device that delivers an electric shock to the heart muscle through the chest wall in order to restore a normal heart rate.

An AED is a portable defibrillator designed to be used by people without substantial medical training who are responding to a cardiac emergency.

Employers have a duty to provide first aid equipment at all places of work where working conditions require it. Depending on the size or specific hazards of the place of work, trained occupational first aiders must also be provided. First aid rooms must be provided where appropriate (e.g. where there are no medical facilities such as those in a hospital).

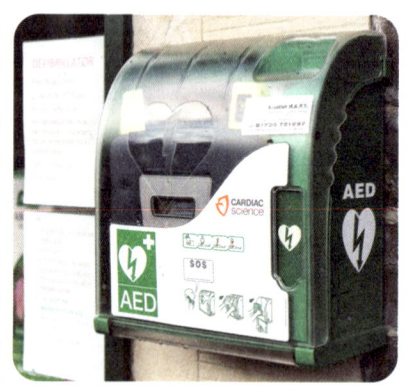

In healthcare environments all nursing staff must participate in cardiopulmonary resuscitation (CPR) courses every two years: this is a mandatory requirement in the HSE, and recommended by the Irish Heart Foundation as good practice. This training equips staff with the skills to remain calm and confident in a life-threatening situation in the knowledge that they are doing the right thing. In other areas of healthcare, training requirements are regulated by local policy.

Safety Signs

Safety signage is obligatory in all workplaces to inform users of or draw their attention to objects and situations capable of causing specific hazards.

(HSA 2007)

Safety signs are short, specific written or pictorial instructions or warnings of hazards. Signs should always be used where a hazard cannot be avoided.

Many signs are internationally recognisable and have no writing on them. Safety signs use standardised shapes and colours to highlight their meaning.

Colours and shapes used for safety signs:

- Red = prohibition
- Yellow = caution
- Green = positive action
- Blue = mandatory actions
- Circles = prohibitions and instructions
- Triangles = warnings
- Squares and rectangles = emergency and information signs.

A safety sign provides information about safety or health and can be a signboard, a colour, acoustic signal, oral communication or hand signal.

A **signboard** provides information using a combination of shape, colour and symbols but no words. However, some signs can be incredibly detailed and generally relate to specific work environments or emergency procedures.

Prohibition signs indicate that certain actions are forbidden. They are circular signs with a black pictogram on a white background with red edging and a diagonal line.

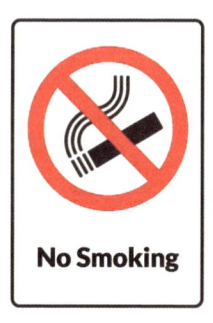

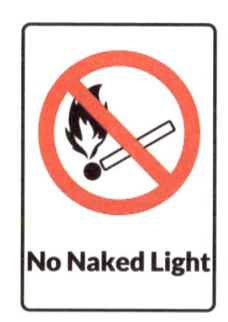

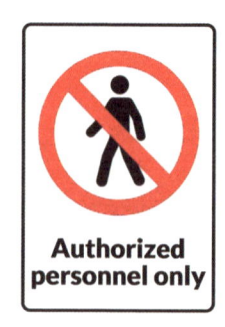

Mandatory signs indicate actions that must be undertaken. They are circular signs with a white pictogram on a blue background.

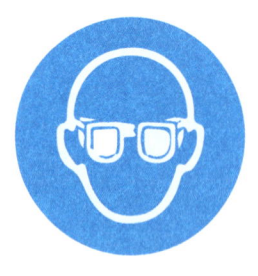

Safety glasses must be worn

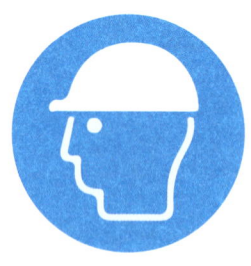

Hard hats must be worn

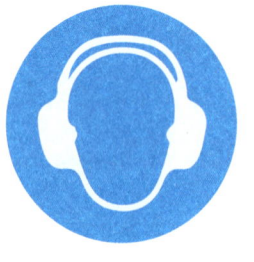

Earmuffs must be worn

Warning signs indicate possible hazards. They are triangular signs with a black pictogram on a yellow background.

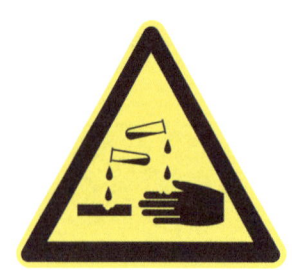

Danger – corrosion risk

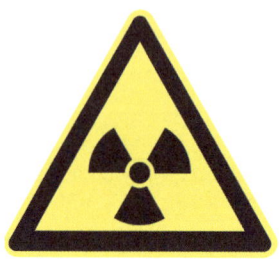

Danger – radiation risk

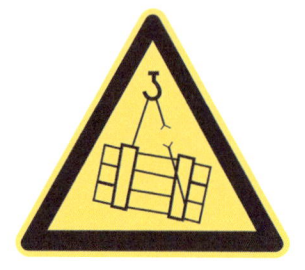

Danger – overhead crane

CHAPTER 08: SAFETY EQUIPMENT

Information signs give information such as the location of rescue equipment, facilities and exits. They are rectangular or square with a white pictogram on a green background.

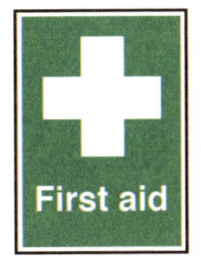

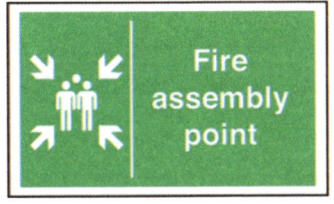

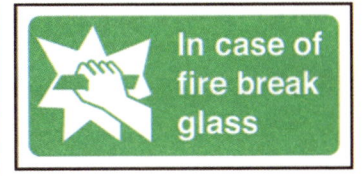

See Appendix 3 for more examples of signs.

chapter 9
COMMUNICATION AND TRAINING

IN THIS CHAPTER YOU WILL LEARN ABOUT:

- The role of communication in promoting health and safety in the workplace
- The role of training in promoting health and safety in the workplace
- Communication across the organisation

Communication and training are essential factors in the promotion and provision of health and safety in the workplace. Safety is everybody's business. The **Safety, Health and Welfare at Work Act 2005 lists specific duties in relation to communication and training: Section 10 deals with training and Section 26 with communication**.

Communication

Good communication is essential to ensure safety in the workplace. It can be examined from three different perspectives:

1. Day-to-day communication with all stakeholders in the healthcare sector – clients, healthcare professionals, supervisors, visitors, contract workers

2. Communication between staff with particular emphasis on handover meetings

3. Communication across the organisation of workplace policies and procedures in accordance with safety and health legislation.

Day-to-day Communication

We use communication every day in nearly every environment, including in the workplace. Communication is simply the transmission of information from one person to another, i.e. sending and receiving messages. In the healthcare sector, we regularly communicate with clients, healthcare professionals, managers and supervisors, and families and friends of our clients. Your role is to determine the needs of your clients and solve their problems in a proactive and pleasant manner; to do this you must be able to communicate effectively with both client and other staff members. It is also your role to ensure that clients' health and well-being is not compromised by your or others' negligence or poor work practices. Safety is not a stand-alone or separate part of your work; it must be central to and immersed in everything you do. Practising the principles of safety is fundamental to providing care and respect for your clients, your colleagues and yourself. It is in everyone's interest to ensure that health and safety is a priority and part of everyday activity in the workplace. This is the message that you communicate by your actions when you practise safety. The verbal messages you communicate are also important, so it is essential that all communication is effective and understood.

(*Skills for Care* 2018)

Barriers to Communication

The individuals you work with or care for may present with barriers to communicating effectively, while aspects of our environment can also create and present barriers.

Some of these barriers are:

+ Speech difficulties due to disabilities or illness, e.g. dementia, stroke
+ Deafness
+ Poor sight
+ Noisy environment – background noise such as machines, loud conversation
+ Poor cognitive skills, e.g. learning disabilities
+ Difference in language spoken
+ Cultural differences
+ Anxiety about a health condition
+ Work overload or time pressures.

Task **Can you think of any other barriers to communication?**

Some tips on how to overcome these barriers include:

+ Use a soft but firm tone of voice
+ Adjust the rate and volume of your speech to suit who you are communicating with
+ Articulate clearly
+ Use rhythm, intonation and stress to get your meaning across
+ Be aware of your facial expression
+ Make eye contact

- Consider using gestures/touch
- Be mindful of your body language and posture
- Ensure client privacy when communicating personal information
- Avoid noisy backgrounds by closing doors/windows and moving away from communal areas.

The Handover Communication

Handovers are an essential part of everyday practice in healthcare and a key part of ensuring client safety. However, many handovers happen at the end of a shift when staff are tired and waiting to go home.

Handover communication is the process of passing client-specific information from one caregiver to another, from one team of caregivers to the next, or from caregivers to the client and family for the purpose of ensuring client care continuity and safety.

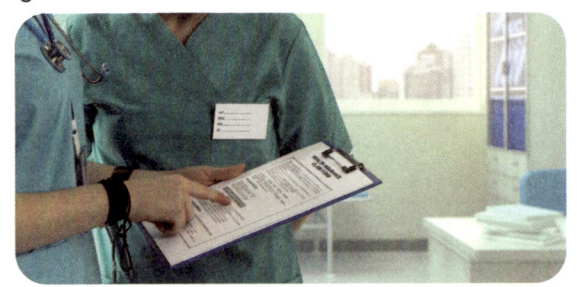

(WHO Joint Commission 2006)

Handover communication also relates to the transfer of information from one type of healthcare organisation to another, or from the healthcare organisation to the client's home. Information shared usually comprises the client's current condition, recent changes in condition, ongoing treatment and possible changes or complications that might occur. Client care handovers occur in many settings across the continuum of care.

During an episode of illness or period of care, a client can potentially be treated by several healthcare practitioners and specialists in multiple settings. Clients will often move between areas of diagnosis, treatment and care and can potentially encounter three shifts of staff each day. Making sure that every handover is done correctly is essential to client safety. Communication between units and between care teams is vital and must include all essential information. It must be clear, unambiguous and leave no room for misunderstanding. Gaps in communication can cause serious breakdowns in the continuity of care, inappropriate treatment and potential harm to the client.

To ensure effective handover communication, the WHO recommends the following:

1. A standardised approach to handover communication between staff, change of shift and between different patient care units in the course of a patient transfer. Suggested elements of this approach include:

    - Use of the SBAR (Situation, Background, Assessment and Recommendation) technique

    - Allocation of sufficient time for communicating important information and for staff to ask and respond to questions without interruptions wherever possible (repeat-back and read-back steps should be included in the handover process)

    - Provision of information regarding the patient's status, medications, treatment plans, advance directives and any significant status changes

    - Limitation of the exchange of information to that which is necessary to providing safe care to the patient.

2. Ensure that healthcare organisations implement systems which ensure that the client and the next healthcare provider are given key information regarding discharge diagnoses, treatment plans, medications and test results.

3. Training on effective handover communication must be an essential part of continuing professional development for healthcare professionals.

4. Communication between organisations that are providing care to the same client in parallel must be encouraged.

(WHO 2007)

Detailed and effective handovers help prepare staff for their shift and to effectively take on the responsibility of the resident's safety. Accurate handovers inform staff of exactly what they need to do and what has arisen in the previous shift or while the staff member was on holiday, such as if a client has missed medication, refused to eat or had a fall; staff can then adjust their care accordingly.

Task Discuss how a poor handover can affect the safety of a client.

Communication across the Organisation

Managing communication of key information on workplace policies and procedures within the organisation is vital. The best policies and procedures are worthless if they are not communicated effectively to all staff/stakeholders: managers, healthcare staff/professionals, employees, clients, their families, visitors and external contractors.

Effective communication is a vital element in the development of a positive safety culture. An effective communication process tells all stakeholders what they need to know in a positive way about health and safety within the workplace. Effective communication is required up, down and across the organisation to achieve success in health and safety.

Decisions on communication plans, including the 'what, who and how', should be part of an overall health and safety strategy. This requires planning, selecting appropriate communication methods and a monitoring system to ensure that the required information is communicated to the required audience in an effective manner that achieves the desired effect.

Poor communication has a number of potentially damaging effects:

- More accidents, injuries and illness
- Reduced productivity and delays
- Risk-taking by employees
- Lack of knowledge regarding legislation
- Higher insurance costs and compensation payouts
- Possible damage to workplace materials and equipment
- Health risks to clients as well as staff.

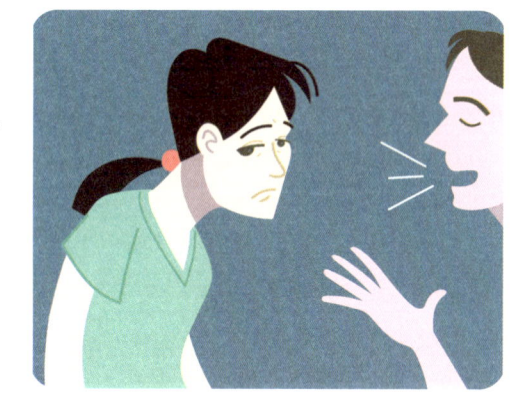

The Importance of Communication in an Organisation

Communication involves building relationships with others, listening and understanding, conveying thoughts and messages clearly and expressing plans coherently and simply. Communication is only successful when the message has been received and the appropriate action taken. The fundamental goal of health and safety communication is to provide meaningful, relevant and accurate information, in clear and understandable terms, to all stakeholders.

Effective communication of health and safety messages:

- Promotes awareness and understanding of the management of health and safety as well as specific risk issues

- Promotes consistency and transparency in health and safety issues and decisions

- Improves the overall effectiveness and efficiency of the health and safety policy and system

- Contributes to the development and delivery of effective and relevant information, instruction and learning opportunities

- Fosters trust and confidence among stakeholders

- Strengthens working relationships

- Supports exchange of information on the knowledge, attitudes, values, practices and perceptions of all stakeholders.

(Croner-i 2020)

Communication Barriers

Barriers to effective communication exist; recognising those barriers and knowing how to overcome them are essential for effective communication. The potential barriers that can hinder effective delivery of a health and safety message are:

- **Information overload:** Too much safety jargon and legalese can obscure the message.

- **Lack of clarity:** The health and safety message should always be clear and concise.

- **Unclear expectations:** Expected results must be clearly defined.

- **Hearing but not listening:** Communication of a safety message without having listened to stakeholders will not be successful. Appropriate stakeholders must fully participate in the communication process.

- **Lack of access to critical data** about health and safety can make effective communication difficult to achieve.

- **Perception differences amongst stakeholders:** Health and safety can mean different things to different people, resulting in messages being perceived in different ways or even ignored.

- **Lack of receptiveness:** Some individuals feel that health and safety is the responsibility of other people.

- **Societal challenges:** These include language differences, cultural factors, religious laws, illiteracy, poverty, a lack of legal, technical and policy resources and a lack of infrastructure that supports communication.

Key Considerations for Effective Communication in Healthcare

Audience. An effective communications system should identify the different groups of people with whom communication is needed, as they may have to be dealt with and approached differently. This includes staff at all levels, clients with different levels of health, infrequent visitors and outside contractors. The message must be clear, concise and capable of being understood by all.

Messages. It is important for an organisation to be consistent so that stakeholders learn to recognise and trust it. Messages may have to be tailored or targeted to various groups to ensure understanding. The information should be objective, clear and as simple as possible.

Messengers. The person(s) delivering the message can have an impact on the delivery of the message. It is important to ensure that the right person delivers the message to the right audience.

Methods. Communication methods should use the most appropriate tools and activities for getting across a particular message. Intranet and email are more likely to be used today than printed newsletters.

Timeline. Communication strategies should include a timeline to ensure that the right messages are delivered at the right time.

Environment. Client privacy must be protected at all times; therefore, it is important when discussing information that may be client-sensitive that it is done privately and never casually in open areas. When communicating directly with a client, ensure that there are no environmental or background interruptions or distractions which may cause misunderstanding or which may lead to a partial message being communicated.

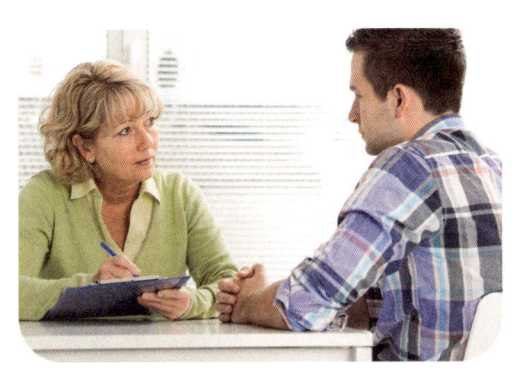

The means by which information is to be communicated at different levels within the organisation should be clear. Effective communication also supports teamwork and co-ordination between groups. Employees learn about, and become part of, an organisation's safety culture through communication.

Ways to communicate your safety message:

+ Send a monthly newsletter via email.

- Put up a noticeboard, either corkboard or electronic, in the canteen or where employees clock in.

- Toolbox talks or routine informal short meetings can cover a different but relevant topic each week/month.

- Safety comment cards puts the onus on employees to report any unsafe acts or safety hazards that they come across.

- Share case studies or incident reports – sharing information about real events and real people is highly effective.

- European Safety Week is run annually and highlights health and safety with many engaging initiatives, such as competitions, information talks, etc.

- Take pictures of safe actions. While it might be tempting to highlight unsafe actions, it is important to promote the positive actions that staff are taking every day to stay safe.

Communication is an essential part of any Health and Safety management system and should include procedures detailing:

- Internal communication at all levels up, down and across the organisation

- Communication with contractors, visitors and other persons allowed in the premises

- How communications from external stakeholders should be received, documented and responded to.

Communication is the key to a healthy, safe and productive workplace. It ensures awareness of health and safety strategies and policies among all staff and it is needed to clearly identify roles and directions; to warn against dangers; to avoid unsafe practices; to promote critical emergency response; and particularly to learn about the concerns and hazards that workers encounter. Communication involves sharing positive messages and when necessary bad news messages; however, the opportunity must always be taken to communicate a bad news message into an undertaking of the organisation's commitment to make changes where needed.

> Effective communication among staff encourages effective teamwork and promotes continuity and clarity within the patient care team. At its best, good communication encourages collaboration, fosters teamwork, and helps prevent errors.
>
> (O'Daniel & Rosenstein 2008)

Task You need to discuss an issue about a resident with a co-worker. Which of these two options is the better approach?

Option 1: You start talking about the issue as soon as you see your co-worker in the hallway.

Option 2: You meet your co-worker in the hallway and ask him when he would be free as you would like to discuss something with him in private.

Training

The **Safety, Health and Welfare at Work Act 2005** strongly advocates providing employees with instruction, information and training necessary to ensure their health and safety. With training, employees acquire the skills, knowledge and attitude to make them competent in the safety and health aspects of their work, which encourages a positive health and safety culture.

Under **Section 10 of the Safety, Health and Welfare at Work Act 2005**, it is the duty of the employer to provide training in a form, manner and language likely to be understood to employees.

Certain conditions and structures must be in place to facilitate training assessment needs and training programmes. Recruitment and placement procedures must ensure that employees are both the most suitable and appropriate candidates for their posts and also those who will find training programmes beneficial. Systems are required to assess and identify training needs as a result of recruitment or changes in staff. Appropriate training documentation must also be considered, to include refresher training where necessary. According to the **2005 Act**, training must be provided to an employee in the following situations:

1. On starting work in the organisation
2. If new processes, equipment or systems of work are introduced which require training, e.g. change to roof hoist
3. On a regular basis as determined by local policy, e.g. HIQA
4. If a risk assessment identifies training as a required control measure, e.g. client handling, sharps training
5. If an employee is transferred or is assigned to new tasks
6. If an inspector from the HSA directs that training be provided
7. Where there is a legal requirement to renew a training programme, e.g. manual handling every two years
8. On the introduction of new work equipment, systems of work or changes in existing work equipment or systems of work
9. On the introduction of new technology.

Healthcare workers can work in a variety of departments within a hospital or care facility, as well as in, for example, MRI clinics, emergency departments, palliative care, maternity care, phlebotomy outpatients, endoscopy and oncology departments. There is a vast range of training available depending on the sector that you choose to work in. Here is some of the more common types of training:

- HIQA Compliance Training
- Recognising and Responding to Challenging Behaviours including Dementia
- Fire Safety Training
- Infection Prevention and Control
- Safeguarding Vulnerable Adults
- Palliative and End of Life Care
- Manual Handling and People Moving and Handling
- Restrictive Practice
- HACCP and Food Safety Training.

(HIQA 2019)

chapter 10
PERSONAL HEALTH IN THE WORKPLACE

IN THIS CHAPTER YOU WILL LEARN ABOUT:

- Promoting safe and healthy working practices in relation to oneself, others and the workplace
- Risk factors in relation to safety, including the effects of medication, drink and drugs
- Risk factors in relation to health, including stress, lifestyle, diet and illness
- The role of diet and exercise in the promotion of good health

Safe and Healthy Working Practices

Health is a balance between the person and his/her environment and focuses on the physical, social and psychological aspects of a person being in a state of equilibrium. Life choices can influence our physical and mental health and it is up to the individual to maintain a healthy, balanced lifestyle. Different factors affect decision-making and our capacity and capability to ensure a healthy lifestyle: age, sex, social class, working and living conditions, income, education, peer group pressure, mental health and access to information.

(DoHC 2000)

The Safety, Health and Welfare at Work Act 2005 outlines the responsibilities of the employer and employee with regard to maintaining a healthy work environment and work practices.

CHAPTER 10: PERSONAL HEALTH IN THE WORKPLACE

The governance structure of an organisation incorporates principles for maintaining a positive safety and healthy culture. Safe work practices fulfil and support the safety, psychological, behavioural and situational needs of clients, relatives and staff.

- Policies relating to staff welfare: dignity at work, anti-bullying, grievance policy
- Policies relating to safety: safety statements, risk assessments, control measures
- Audit programmes which will guide best practice
- The implementation and use of procedural guidelines and standard operating procedures (SOPs).

Everyone within an organisation has a responsibility to work safely so that their own safety and the safety of their colleagues, clients and clients' relatives is maintained. All staff should adopt the safe work practices listed in Chapter 1 (pages 6–8).

A Safety Culture

> The safety culture of an organisation is the product of individual and group values, attitudes, perceptions, competencies, and patterns of behaviour that determine the commitment to, and the style and proficiency of, an organisation's health and safety management. Organisations with a positive safety culture are characterised by communications founded on mutual trust, by shared perceptions of the importance of safety and by confidence in the efficacy of preventive measures.
>
> (ACSNI 1993)

Key Aspects of Effective Culture

+ **Management commitment:** Active involvement of senior management sets an example of how important health and safety is within the organisation. It becomes an unconscious element of day-to-day operations.

+ **Visible management:** Managers need to be seen to lead by example when it comes to health and safety. Their commitment needs to be visible as well as their actions to support health and safety.

+ **Good communications between all levels of employee:** Messages should be clear, consistent and continuous. Safety and health should be part of daily conversations.

+ **Active employee participation in safety:** Builds ownership of safety at all levels and exploits the unique knowledge that employees have of their own work.

(HSE website: 'Safety Culture')

Promoting an Open and Just Safety Culture

When investigating the circumstances of an incident, the employer must:

1. Interview all staff involved
2. Ensure the client has been reviewed by the medical team and relevant action taken
3. Inform the client of the incident and apologise
4. Organise counselling for the staff involved and identify any training needs
5. Ensure that policies, procedures and guidelines are up to date and all staff are informed.

Encourage a 'See, Sort it' mentality!

Safe Working Environments

There are many safety issues to be considered in the healthcare setting. Continuous monitoring of the work environment to identify hazards or potential hazards must be a high priority and must always be included in any risk assessment.

The employee also has a responsibility to be vigilant and should take personal responsibility for identifying potential or existing hazards and act accordingly to prevent injury.

Role of the employer:

- Provide a safety statement
- Organise safe systems of work (policies, procedures and guidelines)
- Provide appropriate personal protective clothing
- Provide a secure environment for clients' relatives and staff (e.g. adequately lit car parks, secure doors)
- Ensure effective communication strategies (imparting and receiving information)
- Provide training (e.g. manual handling, sharps awareness, clinical waste management)
- Plan for emergencies and provide emergency plans (fire, major incident).

Role of the employee:

- Act appropriately and responsibly, with due care
- Attend training with due regard
- Adhere to safe systems of work (e.g. wearing PPE)

- Identify and act when hazards are identified (dealing with spills straight away, removing broken equipment)
- Adhere to best practice (policies, procedures and guidelines)
- Apply principles of good housekeeping (prevention of slips, trips and falls)
- Wear name badge
- Manage waste according to local policy
- Report incidents (e.g. report equipment defects and document event).

Reducing Workplace Accidents and Incidents

The following standardised research-based work practices are considered effective in reducing the number of adverse events and incidences in an organisation:

1. Being consistent in work practice
2. Following recommended standard operating procedures
3. Provision of training
4. Attendance at training, with due regard.

The main aim of any organisation is to make sure that no one gets hurt or becomes ill. Accidents and ill health can ruin lives, and can also affect business if output is lost, equipment is damaged, insurance costs increase, or if a claim is made and there is a court case. Carrying out risk assessments, preparing and implementing a safety statement and keeping both up to date will not in themselves prevent accidents and ill health but they will play a crucial part in reducing the likelihood of them happening.

Management Role in Managing Risk

Employers, managers and supervisors have key responsibilities in the management of risk. They should all ensure that workplace practices reflect the risk assessments and safety statement. This can be achieved by:

- Ensuring that behaviour at work reflects the safe working practices laid down in these documents
- Carrying out supervisory checks and audits to determine how well the aims set down are being achieved
- Take corrective action when required.

Additionally, if a workplace is provided for use by others, the safety statement must set out the safe work practices that are relevant to them.

We have already seen that the **Safety, Health and Welfare at Work Act 2005 requires employers to identify hazards, carry out a risk assessment and prepare a written safety statement**. This process helps employers and unit/ward managers to manage employees' safety and health and get the balance right between the seriousness of any safety and health problems and what must be done about them. The system must involve consultation between the employer and employees, who are required by law to co-operate with the employer in the safety management process.

All employees and external contractors must pay due regard to all the safety processes in the organisation. The most important documentation to enable employees to achieve this is the safety statement, together with supporting policies, procedures and guidelines. The employer must ensure that the safety statement, which includes risk assessments, is brought to the attention of all employees and others at the workplace who may be exposed to any risks covered by the safety statement. All new employees must be made aware of the safety statement when they start work. The statement must be in a form and language that they all understand.

External Contractors

In addition to the organisation's employees, other people may be exposed to a specific risk dealt with in the safety statement and the statement should be brought to their attention.

These people could include:

- Outside contractors who do cleaning, maintenance or building work
- Temporary workers
- Delivery people who stack their goods in the premises and come into contact with activities there
- Self-employed people who provide a service for the organisation.

Where specific tasks pose a serious risk to safety and health, the relevant contents of the safety statement must be brought to the attention of those affected, setting out the hazards identified, the risk assessments and the safety and health measures that must be taken.

Risk Factors in Relation to Health

There are many risk factors in relation to health for healthcare workers, such as smoking, alcohol, diet, drugs, injury from exercise, sexual health and stress.

Each of these factors can compromise a person's health and ability to function safely in the workplace.

Lifestyle

People make choices that affect how they live their lives. Everyone needs to take personal responsibility to ensure the choices they make are in their own best interest. Education and health promotion can inform employees of the positive choices to maintain a healthy work/life balance. However, an individual must be ready to make those changes for themselves, which includes making positive choices in relation to their lifestyle and diet in order to reduce the risk of illness. Excessive use of or dependence on alcohol, drugs or smoking will have a detrimental effect on health, and cause a deterioration in a person's ability to function optimally. Sub-standard performance at work leaves the worker and those around them open to greater incident of risk.

Poor lifestyle choices can lead to:

- Tiredness
- Poor attendance
- Illness/absence
- Lack of concentration
- Poor morale
- Lethargy
- Lack of motivation.

When an employee exhibits any of these symptoms it can severely impact on the safety, health and welfare of clients, relatives and other employees. It also has a negative impact on the performance and productivity of an organisation.

Stress

Stress is a natural reaction to excessive pressure. It can be work-related or due to personal circumstances. Work-related stress occurs when work demands do not match a person's knowledge, skill and/or ability.

Work-based stress can be caused by:

- Excessive demands caused by a change in workload
- Change of work patterns
- Lack of support
- Conflict with colleagues
- Unclear roles
- Lack of recognition.

Symptoms of stress

Physical	Psychological
Raised heart rate	Heightened emotional state
Increased respiration rate	Feelings of being overpowered
Dry mouth	Fear
Sweaty palms	Feelings of loss of control
Digestive upset	

Organisational Effects of Stress

When employees are stressed, work performance is impaired, which in turn can affect productivity. An employee may display behaviours such as poor time-keeping, absenteeism and poor concentration.

Employers have a responsibility under the **Safety, Health and Welfare at Work Act 2005** to:

- Raise awareness
- Communicate the organisation's commitment to tackling stress
- Provide a support structure for staff
- Ensure clear roles and responsibilities
- Ensure appropriate procedures are in place to deal with bullying, complaints, violence and aggression
- Protect vulnerable groups such as pregnant employees or disabled employees.

Diet and Exercise

To help maintain health, an individual should eat a balanced diet. The food pyramid identifies the proportion of protein, fat and carbohydrates a person should eat every day. Healthy eating is about getting the correct amount of nutrients – protein, fat, carbohydrates, vitamins and minerals – needed to maintain good health.

Foods that contain the same type of nutrients are grouped together on the shelves of the food pyramid. This gives you a choice of different foods from which to choose a healthy diet. Following the food pyramid as a guide will help you get the right balance of nutritious foods within your calorie range.

Studies show that we take in too many calories from foods and drinks high in fat, sugar and salt (on the top shelf of the food pyramid). These provide very little of the essential vitamins and minerals our body needs. Limiting these is essential for healthy eating.

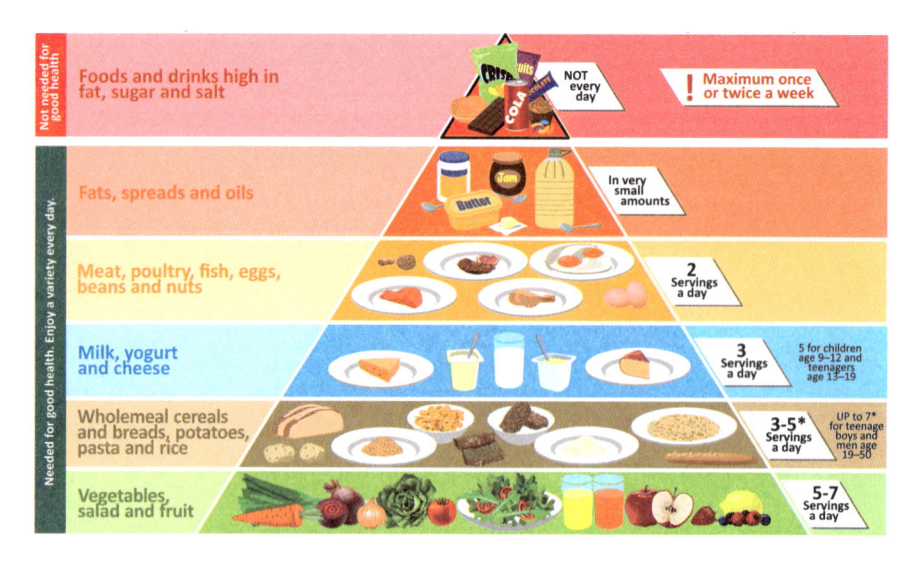

(Irish Institute of Nutrition and Health (IINH) https://www.iinh.net/new-food-pyramid-2016/)

Eating healthily helps maintain a good nutritional balance, and eating the recommended portion sizes of good-quality food will help regulate the metabolism.

Healthy eating involves:

- Bread, rice, potatoes, pasta and cereals – going for the wholegrain varieties whenever you can
- Fruit and vegetables
- Some milk, cheese and yoghurt
- Some meat, poultry, eggs, beans and nuts
- A very small amount of fats and oils
- A very small amount or no food and drinks high in fat, sugar and salt.

The benefits of maintaining a healthy diet are:

- Reduced risk of stroke and other cardiovascular diseases
- Reduced risk of type 2 diabetes
- Protection against certain cancers, such as mouth, stomach and colon-rectum cancer
- Reduced risk of coronary artery disease
- Decreased bone loss
- Reduced risk of developing kidney stones.

Exercise

Regular physical activity is one of the most important things you can do for your health. It is recommended that a person should take 30 minutes of moderate to intensive exercise at least five times per week, every week.

The benefits of regular physical activity include:

- Helps to control weight
- Reduces the risk of cardiovascular disease
- Reduces the risk of type 2 diabetes and metabolic syndrome
- Reduces the risk of some cancers
- Strengthens bones and muscles
- Improves mental health and mood
- Improves ability to do daily activities and helps prevent falls (older adults)
- Increases your chances of living longer
- Increases energy

- Reduces stress
- Improves sleep patterns.

Promoting Safety and Health in the Workplace

To create and promote a safety culture within an organisation, it is essential that management:

- Enable employees to be proactive on safety and health
- Motivate employees on safety and health
- Reward good safety and health practices
- Make sure all employees understand their safety and health roles
- Facilitate the safety representative role
- Use the safety committee to promote safety and health excellence
- Engage with employees on developing safe procedures
- Encourage progress and programmes for improvement
- Promote positive safety and health feedback.

Experience has shown that positive employee engagement reaps dividends and ensures greater safety and health compliance. **Section 26 of the 2005 Act** provides for consultation between employers and employees to help ensure co-operation in preventing accidents and ill health. Under **Section 25 of the 2005 Act**, employees are entitled to select a safety representative to represent them on safety and health matters with their employer. Section 26 sets out the arrangements for this consultation on a range of safety and health issues in the workplace. Where a safety committee is in existence in a workplace, it can be used for this consultation process. These are key provisions of the **2005 Act** and a central part of the preventive system of promoting safety and health at work. Managers must enable all employees to engage in safety and health promotion. It is essential that all employees know and understand their role and realise that they are agents for promoting better safety and health.

The best way to get workers to follow safe procedures and systems is for them to be involved in developing and reviewing those systems. If people feel that their opinions are valued and considered, they are much more likely to follow the processes when they are implemented. It is critical to get the right people involved at the right time; the people who are doing the job know that job better than anyone. Given the right approach and opportunity, workers will let managers know the correct way to do a job, and if they are encouraged to contribute in this way they are also extremely likely to work in the correct way.

A positive safety and health culture increase safety and health compliance. A safety and health culture is the product of the individual and group values, attitudes, perceptions, competencies and patterns of behaviour. If these elements are in place and all other factors are right in the workplace, then the compliance standards will be strictly adhered to by all. Creating a positive safety and health culture in the workplace means ensuring the correct standards and procedures are in place and that workers comply with these standards.

(HSA n.d.)

Active-effective listening and clear instructions contribute to a positive health and safety culture. Indicators of a positive safety culture are:

- Strong leadership
- Two-way communication

- Staff involvement
- Existence of a learning and just culture.

Reducing Risk in the Workplace: Employees' Responsibilities

All employees must come to work free from the effects of any intoxicant, e.g. alcohol, drugs.

Section 13 (1) (b) of the 2005 Act states:

> Any Employee, while at work, must ensure that he or she is not under the influence of an intoxicant where the extent of the intoxication could endanger his or her own safety, health, or welfare at work or that of any other person present. In the event an employer has concerns that an employee is acting inappropriately or is a danger to himself/herself or others the correct action is to remove that employee from the situation. In the event an employee's behaviour is such that he/she is a danger to him/herself and is removed from the situation, the employer has a duty of care to that employee and can suggest that this person avail of the support systems within the organisation, e.g. counselling, access to the Occupational Health service.

Examples of intoxicants (legal and illegal) include:

- Alcohol
- Cannabis
- Cocaine
- All classifications of banned substances

- Prescribed medicines (which can influence a person's ability to carry out their task safely).

Excessive consumption of medication, alcohol or drugs can have a range of negative health effects, including:

- Dizziness
- High blood pressure
- Low blood pressure
- Fatigue
- Stress
- Aggression
- Liver disease
- Heart disease
- Mental health issues.

As employees in healthcare, we also need to be mindful and vigilant when caring for clients to ensure that best practice is adhered to regarding medication management. As a carer, you will not be dispensing medication, but you may be asked to assist the nurse, e.g. removing a nebuliser mask, assisting in positioning a client for medication to be administered. Safety is everyone's business. It is essential as a front-line carer to report any changes observed in the client, e.g. episodes of drowsiness or confusion, as this may be an indication of medication error.

GLOSSARY OF HEALTH AND SAFETY TERMS

Accident - An undesired, unplanned incident resulting in injury, ill-health, death or damage.

Airborne - particles (aerosols) Very small particles that may contain infectious agents. They can remain in the air for long periods of time and can be carried over long distances by air currents.

Alcohol based hand rub - A gel, foam or liquid containing one or more types of alcohol that is rubbed into the hands to inactivate microorganisms and/or temporarily suppress their growth.

Allergen - A substance that causes an allergic reaction in the body.

Antibiotic - A substance that kills or inhibits the growth of bacteria.

Asbestos - The name used for a group of fibrous silicate minerals that once inhaled, have adverse effects on health and can lead to fatal lung diseases.

Audit - An official inspection of the health and safety management arrangements of a premises, carried out by qualified auditors. The aim of an audit is to confirm that adequate control measures have been put in place to cover the risks and to ensure that these measures are being adhered to.

Best Practice - A standard of risk control that is above the legal minimum.

Blood Borne Viruses (BBV) - Viruses carried or transmitted by blood, for example Hepatitis B, Hepatitis C and HIV.

Clostridioides difficile (C.diff) - An infectious agent (bacterium) that can cause mild to severe diarrhoea which in some cases can lead to gastro-intestinal complications and death.

Compliance - The act or process of fulfilling requirements.

Corrosive - A substance that has destructive effects on another substance.

Fires -
  Class A: Fires with flammable solids such as wood, plastic and paper.
  Class B: Fires involving flammable liquids and electrical fires.
  Class C: Fires involving gases.
  Class D: Fires involving metals such as magnesium, potassium and titanium.
  Class F: Fires with cooking oils and fats.

First Aid - The skilled application of accepted principles of treatment on the occurrence of an accident or in the case of sudden illness, using facilities or materials available at the time.

Flammable Gas - A gas with a low flammability limit that can be readily ignited when mixed with air.

Flammable Liquid - A liquid which can readily catch fire.

Flammable Solid - Solids that are liable to cause fires through friction or absorption of moisture.

Hazard - A potential source of harm.

Incident - A term for those events that have not resulted in significant harm but have the potential to cause an accident, injury or damage under different circumstances.

Irritant - A non-corrosive substance which can cause inflammation on the body through contact.

Manual Handling - Any means of transporting or supporting a load manually. Lifting, putting down, pushing, pulling, carrying or moving by hand or bodily force.

Material Data Safety Sheet - A document that details information on potentially hazardous substances, along with guidance on how to handle them safely.

Risk Assessment - An examination of the potential risks in the workplace, with the aim of assessing whether enough precautions have been put in place to prevent harm. A risk assessment focuses on the relationship between the worker, the work being carried out, the equipment being used and the conditions of the working environment.

Safe Systems of Work - A method of working designed to eliminate, if possible, or otherwise reduce risks to health and safety.

Toxic Substances - Substances that cause irritation or are otherwise harmful to health, such as carcinogens and poisons.

Vapour - The gaseous form of a substance that is normally liquid or solid at room temperature.

APPENDICES

appendix 1
SAMPLE ACCIDENT/INCIDENT REPORT FORM

ACCIDENT/INCIDENT REPORT FORM

This form should be completed by the Supervisor/Manager and returned to the Safety Officer and/or HR Office.

Name of Injured Person _____

Date & Time of Accident/Incident _____

Employee [ ]   Other [ ]

Exact Location of the Accident/Incident (Work Area)
_____

Type of activity taking place at the time:
_____

What activity was the injured person involved in?
_____

Were others carrying out the same activity?
_____

Name of the Supervisor when the accident took place:
_____

Give a full description of accident/incident/damage to property, etc:
_____
_____

First aid/medical care following the accident/incident (e.g. first aider, doctor, ambulance)
_____

Describe actions taken to prevent the accident/incident happening again:
_____

Details of the injury:

Infection _____   Bruising _____

Fracture _____   Open wound _____

Head injury _____   Sprain/torn ligaments _____

Poisoning _____   Burns/scalding _____

Other _____

Did injured person:

Go home [ ]   Visit doctor [ ]   Go to A&E [ ]   Stay in hospital [ ]

Tick if out of work with the injury:

0 days [ ]   1–3 days [ ]   4–7 days [ ]   7+ days [ ]

Signed _____   Signed _____

Date _____   Date _____

Supervisor/Manager   Safety Officer

appendix 2
SAMPLE OF COMPLETED RISK ASSESSMENT: SLIPS, TRIPS AND FALLS

Step 1: Identify Hazards	Step 2: Assessing the Risks			Step 3: Additional Control Measures (further actions needed)		
What are the hazards?	Who is at risk?	Current controls (What are you already doing?)	Level of risk? (Your estimate of the remaining risk level, based on the current controls, for example High, Medium, or Low)	Additional controls needed (Further action to reduce the remaining risk level to as low as possible)	Action by whom and by when?	Date completed
Slips, Trips and Falls Can cause serious injuries, for example fractures, head injuries	Everyone – employees and visitors	Clear, unobstructed, slip-resistant pedestrian routes (including entrances and exits) are provided and maintained	Medium	Changes in levels are avoided if possible or are adequately highlighted where necessary – steps outside the side entrance are dark and hard to see	John Smith by August 2018	
		Adequate lighting is provided and is appropriate for the work being carried out				
		Absorbent materials and warning signage are available for dealing with spills				
		Spills are cleaned up immediately		Trailing cables and leads are re-routed, removed or secured – not done in the main office	John Smith by 30 June 2018	
		Mats are properly located, fitted and secured				
		Good housekeeping practices are in place and are maintained				
		Slip-resistant footwear is provided and worn by kitchen staff				

Risk Assessment Completed By: Joe Murphy   Date: 28 June 2018

(HSA 2016a.)

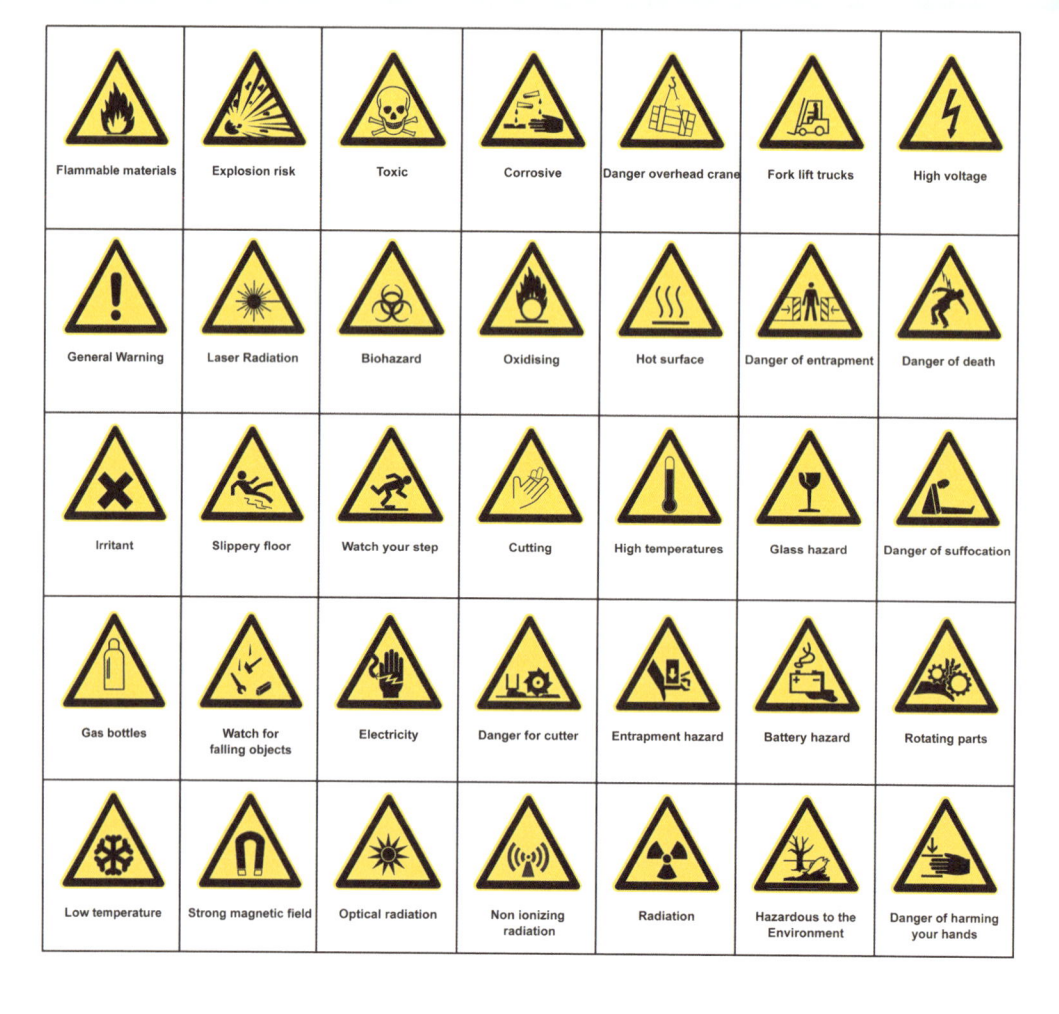

appendix 3
HAZARD SIGNS

Flammable materials	Explosion risk	Toxic	Corrosive	Danger overhead crane	Fork lift trucks	High voltage	
General Warning	Laser Radiation	Biohazard	Oxidising	Hot surface	Danger of entrapment	Danger of death	
Irritant	Slippery floor	Watch your step	Cutting	High temperatures	Glass hazard	Danger of suffocation	
Gas bottles	Watch for falling objects	Electricity	Danger for cutter	Entrapment hazard	Battery hazard	Rotating parts	
Low temperature	Strong magnetic field	Optical radiation	Non ionizing radiation	Radiation	Hazardous to the Environment	Danger of harming your hands	

REFERENCES AND FURTHER READING

ACSNI Human Factors Study Group (1993) *Organising for Safety* (Third Report). HSE Books.

CDCP (Centers for Disease Control and Prevention) 'About Parasites' <https://www.cdc.gov/parasites/about.html> .

CDCP (website) <https://www.cdc.gov/hai/infectiontypes.html>.

Cowan, J. P. (1994) *Handbook of Environmental Acoustics*. Indiana: Van Nostrand Reinhold.

Croner-i (2020) 'Health and Safety Communication Strategies'. London. <https://app.croneri.co.uk/feature-articles/health-and-safety-communication-strategies>.

CSO (Central Statistics Office) (2019) 'Employment (ILO) (Thousand) by NACE Rev 2 Economic Sector' <https://statbank.cso.ie/multiquicktables/quickTables.aspx?id=qlf03>.

DoHC (Department of Health and Children) (2000) *Our Children – Their Lives*. Dublin: Stationery Office.

DoHC (2004) 'Segregation, Packaging and Storage Guidelines for Healthcare Risk Waste'. Dublin.

EASHW (European Agency for Safety and Health at Work) (2002) 'Work-related Stress' (Factsheet 22). Belgium. <https://osha.europa.eu/en/publications/factsheets/22>.

EASHW (2011) 'Innovative Solutions to Safety and Health Risks in the Construction, Healthcare and HORECA Sectors'. Luxembourg.

ESRI (Economic and Social Research Institute) (2015) 'Job Stress and Working Conditions: Ireland in Comparative Perspective: An Analysis of the European Working Conditions Survey' (Research Series No. 84: Helen Russell, Bertrand Maître, Dorothy Watson, Eamonn Fahey). Dublin.

ESRI (2018) 'Trends and Patterns in Occupational Health and Safety in Ireland' (Research Series No. 40: Helen Russell, Bertrand Maître, Dorothy Watson). Dublin.

HIQA (Health Information and Quality Authority) (2016) 'Fire Precautions in Designated Centres for Older People' <https://www.hiqa.ie/sites/default/files/2017-01/Guidance-on-Fire-Compliance-for-Designated-Centres-Older-People.pdf> accessed 16 February 2020.

HIQA (2019) 'National Standards and Guidance' <https://www.hiqa.ie/areas-we-work/standards-and-quality>.

HPSC (Health Protection Surveillance Centre) (website) <https://www.hpsc.ie/a-z/respiratory/coronavirus/novelcoronavirus/guidance/guidanceforhealthcareworkers>.

HSA (Health and Safety Authority) (website) 'Biological Agents' <https://www.hsa.ie/eng/Topics/Biological_Agents>.

HSA 'Emergency Escape and Fire Fighting' <https://www.hsa.ie/eng/Topics/Fire/Emergency_Escape_and_Fire_Fighting/#eva>.

HSA 'Fire Prevention' <https://www.hsa.ie/eng/Topics/Fire/Fire_Prevention/>.

HSA 'PPE – FAQs' <https://www.hsa.ie/eng/Topics/Personal_Protective_Equipment_-_PPE/PPE_-FAQs/Personal_Protective_Equipment_FAQ_Responses.html#PPE>.

HSA <https://www.hsa.ie/eng/Your_Industry/Healthcare_Sector/Electricity_and_Healthcare>.

HSA 'Prevention of Glove-related Latex Allergy in Healthcare Workers' <https://www.hsa.ie/eng/Your_Industry/Healthcare_Sector/Latex_Gloves_Information_Sheet.pdf>.

HSA (n.d.) 'A Guide to Managing Best Practices in Safety and Health'. Dublin. <https://www.hsa.ie/eng/Publications_and_Forms/Publications/Safety_and_Health_Management/Best_Practices_in_Safety_Guide.pdf>.

HSA (2001) 'Report of the Advisory Committee on Health Services'. Dublin.

HSA (2005) 'A Short Guide to the Safety, Health and Welfare at Work Act 2005'. Dublin.

HSA (2007) 'Guide to the Safety, Health and Welfare at Work (General Application) Regulations 2007: Chapter 1 of Part 6: Protection of Children and Young Persons'. Dublin. <https://www.hsa.ie/eng/Publications_and_Forms/Publications/Retail/Gen_Apps_Children_Young_Persons.pdf>.

HSA (2008) 'Guidelines On Occupational Asthma'. Dublin.

HSA (2010) 'Health and Safety Management in Healthcare' Information Sheet. Dublin.

HSA (2011a) 'Guidance on Lone Working in the Healthcare Sector'. Dublin.

HSA (2011b) 'Guidance on the Management of Manual Handling in Healthcare'. Dublin.

HSA (2011c) 'Guidance on Safety with Mobile Patient Hoists and Slings in Healthcare Establishments' Information Sheet. Dublin.

HSA (2012a) 'Guidance for Employers and Employees on Night and Shift Work'. HSA, Dublin.

HSA (2012b) 'Health and Safety at Work in Residential Care Facilities'. Dublin.

HSA (2014) 'Managing the Risk of Work-related Violence and Aggression in Healthcare' Information Sheet. Dublin.

HSA (2016a) 'A Guide to Risk Assessments and Safety Statements'. Dublin.

HSA (2016b) 'Guidance on the Safety, Health and Welfare at Work (Reporting of Accidents and Dangerous Occurrences) Regulations 2016'. Dublin. <https://www.hsa.ie/eng/Publications_and_Forms/Publications/Safety_and_Health_Management/Accident_and_Dangerous_Occurrences_Reporting.pdf>.

HSA (2016c) 'HSA Guide to the Safety, Health and Welfare at Work (General Application) Regulations 2007 Chapter 1 of Part 7: Safety Signs at Places of Work (Amended 2016)'. Dublin.

HSA (2017) 'Occupational Safety and Health and Home Care'. Dublin.

HSA (2019) Strategic Statement 2019-21, Dublin. <https://www.hsa.ie/eng/publications_and_forms/publications/corporate/hsa_strategy_statement_2019-21.pdf>.

HSA (2019a) 'Summary of Workplace Injury, Illness and Fatality Statistics 2017–2018' <https://www.hsa.ie/eng/publications_and_forms/publications/corporate/hsa_stats_report_2019.pdf>.

HSA (2019b) 'Safety Statement' <https://www.hsa.ie/eng/Topics/Managing_Health_and_Safety/Safety_Statement_and_Risk_Assessment/> accessed 1 March 2020.

Health Services Executive (HSE) 'Health and Safety Legislation' <https://www.hse.ie/eng/staff/safetywellbeing/healthsafetyand%20wellbeing/healthandsafetylegislation.html>.

Health and Safety Executive UK 'Safety Culture' (Common Topics: Topic 4) <https://www.hse.gov.uk/humanfactors/topics/common4.pdf>.

HSE (2008) 'Guidelines on Occupational Asthma'. Dublin. <https://www.hsa.ie/eng/Publications_and_Forms/Publications/Occupational_Health/Guidelines_on_Occupational_Asthma.pdf>.

HSE (2011) 'Quality and Patient Safety' <http://www.hse.ie/eng/about/Who/qualityandpatientsafety/resourcesintelligence/Quality_and_Patient_Safety_Documents/riskoctober.pdf> accessed 7 March 2020.

HSE (2012) Patient Safety Toolbox Talks <https://www.hse.ie/eng/about/who/qid/resourcespublications/tool-box-talks/infection-prevention-and-control-sharps-injury.pdf>.

HSE (2015) 'Safety Advisory/Guidance Note: Preventing Slips, Trips and Falls (STFs)'. Dublin. <https://www.hse.ie/eng/staff/safetywellbeing/healthsafetyand%20wellbeing/stfsagn.pdf>.

HSE (2018) 'Policy for Prevention and Management of Stress in the Workplace 2018'. Dublin. <https://www.hse.ie/eng/staff/safetywellbeing/healthsafetyand%20wellbeing/policy%20for%20prevention%20and%20management%20of%20stress%20in%20the%20workplace%202018.pdf>.

HSE (2020) 'Public Health Guidelines on the Prevention and Management of Influenza Outbreaks in Residential Care Facilities in Ireland 2019/2020', Public Health Medicine Communicable Disease Group <https://www.hpsc.ie/a-z/respiratory/influenza/seasonalinfluenza/guidance/residentialcarefacilitiesguidance/Management%20ILI%20and%20influenza%20in%20residential%20care%20facilities.pdf>.

Hughes, R. (2013) '10 Signs an Employee may be Suffering from Stress and Anxiety'. British Association for Counselling and Psychotherapy (BACP).

Joint Commission (2006) 'National Patient Safety Goal FAQs'. Joint Commission, Oakbrook Terrace, IL <https://www.jointcommission.

org/-/media/deprecated-unorganized/imported-assets/tjc/system-folders/topics-library/psc_for_webpdf.pdf?db=web&hash=1D79BF046A319BE99A20BE459982387>.

Joseph, A. and Ulrich, R. (2007) 'Sound Control for Improved Outcomes in Healthcare Settings' <https://www.healthdesign.org/sites/default/files/Sound%20Control.pdf> accessed 16 January 2020.

Mayo Clinic (2019) 'Occupational Asthma', <https://www.mayoclinic.org/diseases-conditions/occupational-asthma/symptoms-causes/syc-20375772> accessed 27 March 2020.

NIFAST (2015) *Safety and Health at Work*. Gill & Macmillan, Dublin.

O'Daniel, M. and Rosenstein, A.H. (2008) 'Professional Communication and Team Collaboration', Chapter 33 in R.G. Hughes (ed.), *Patient Safety and Quality: An Evidence-Based Handbook for Nurses*. Rockville (MD): Agency for Healthcare Research and Quality.

Oireachtas (2005) Safety, Health and Welfare at Work Act 2005 <https://www.irishstatutebook.ie>.

Skills for Care (2018) 'Communication Skills in Social Care' <https://www.skillsforcare.org.uk/Documents/Learning-and-development/Core-skills/Communication-skills-in-social-care.pdf> accessed 18 November 2019.

Stoewen, Debbie L. (2016) 'Wellness at Work: Building Healthy Workplaces', *Canadian Veterinary Journal*, 57(11), 1188–90. Available at: <https://www.ncbi.nlm.nih.gov/pmc/articles/PMC5081153/>.

WHO (World Health Organization) 'Coronavirus' <https://www.who.int/health-topics/coronavirus#tab=tab_1>.

WHO (2010a) 'Healthy Workplaces: A Model for Action for Employers, Workers, Policy-makers and Practitioners' <https://www.who.int/occupational_health/publications/healthy_workplaces_model_action.pdf> accessed 27 December 2019.

WHO (2010b) 'Healthy Workplace Framework and Model: Background and Supporting Literature and Practices' (Joan Burton). Switzerland. <https://www.who.int/occupational_health/healthy_workplace_framework.pdf>.

WHO (2016) 'Worklace Health Promotion' <http://www.who.int/occupational_health/topics/workplace/en/index1.html> accessed 4 March 2020.

WHO Joint Commission (2007) 'Communicating During Patient Hand-Overs', *Patient Safety Solutions*, Vol. 1, Solution 3, May. <https://www.who.int/patientsafety/solutions/patientsafety/PS-Solution3.pdf>.

Answers to quiz in Chapter 1:

1 False

2 False

3 True

4 True

INDEX

A
Accident investigations 26
Accidents 13 16 20–26 31 32 45 142 154 162
Active monitoring 15
AED Automated External Defibrillator 132
Alarm system 22 90 93 94
Alcohol 8 57 156 157 164 165
Audit 16 40 42 151 155
Automated External Defibrillator see AED 132

B
Bacteria 98–105 111
Biological hazards 50 58–62
   Non-risk waste 59
   Risk waste 59
   Safe disposal of sharps 63–64
   Sharps 62
Blood-borne diseases 64 109 111 113
   Hepatitis B 64 100 103 111 112 166
   Hepatitis C 64 100 103 111 112 166

C
Cancer 26 109 111 114 161
Chain of infection 106–108 116

Chemical Hazards 35 50 52
   Disinfecting 52
   Sterilising agent 52
Chemical spillage 26
Communication 21 22 76 133 136–149 153 163
   Communication in organisations 141–143
   Barriers to 143–144
   Day-to-day communication 137
   barriers to 137
   handover communication 139–141
Compartmentation 90
CORU 5
Covid-19 100 114
Crash mats 51
Cytotoxic drugs 52 61
   Absorption 52
   Ingestion 53
   Inhalation 52
   Inoculation 53

D
Decibels 68
Dental Council of Ireland 5
Dermatitis 71–73
Dignity 151
Disabled employees 159

Diseases 24 26 32 102 161
Doors 84 90 91 93 119 139 153

E
Electrical equipment 34 78–79 82 86
Electrical safety rules 79
Emergency escape 82 92
Emergency plans 21 22 53 81 91 153
Emergency procedures 13 22 40 65 66 91 115 133
Employees' duties 8
  Emergency plans 21
  Fire drills 23
  Intoxicants 164
  PPE use 124
  Safety processes 155
  Safety statement 10–12
Employers' duties 5–7
  Duty of care 164
  Healthy work environment 150–153
  Lone workers 44
  Manual handling 75
  Night shift workers 46
  PPE 122–123
  Risk Assessment 29 30 32
  Safety Statement 10–12 41–43
  Training 148
  Young workers 46–47
Ergonomic conditions 75
Escape routes 89 93

F
Fatal injuries 24
Fire blankets 86 88 89
Fire brigade 93 94

Fire classification 87
Fire door 90
Fire evacuation procedures 89–93
Fire-fighting checklist 92
Fire-fighting equipment 86–88
Fire prevention 78–97
Fire triangle 82–83
First aid kit 129–130
  Contents of 130–131
Food pyramid 159–160
Food Safety Authority of Ireland 5
Footwear 19 39 51 128
FSAI see Food Safety Authority of Ireland 5
Fuel 82 83 84 85 86
Fungi 98 99 101

G
Gardaí 24
Gases 52 70 88 167
  Anaesthetic gases 52
  Medical gases 52
Good housekeeping 16–20
  Benefits of 20
  Five Ss of 17
  Procedures 18

H
Hand washing 73
Handling foul/infected linen 120
Handover Communication 139–141
Hazards 7 10 11 15 29 30 31 33 34
  Biological hazards 58–62
  Chemical hazard 35 50 52
  Health Hazards 34–35
  Human Factor Hazards 35
  Physical hazard 34 50–52
  Psychosocial hazards 53–58

Health and Safety Authority (HSA) 3–4
Health and Social Care Professionals Council (CORU) 5
Health and Information Quality Authority (HIQA) 5
Health Products Regulatory Authority 5
Healthcare Associated Infections (HCAIs) 108–113
   Clostridium Difficile 110
   HIV 112–113
   Legionnaire's Disease 111
   MRSA 109
   Norovirus 110
   Tuberculosis 113
Healthcare linen 108 119
   handling clean linen 119
   handling dirty linen 119–120
   handling of foul infected linen 120–121
   storage of clean linen 119
Healthcare waste 59–60
   Disposal of 60
Healthy diet 159
   Benefits of 161
Healthy eating 159
Hierarchy of control 38–40
   Control measures 30 37 38–40
   Chance 30
   Severity 30 35 36
   Risk 30
HIQA, see Health Information Quality Authority 5
HIV, see Human Immunodeficiency Virus 112–113
HPRB, see Health Products Regulatory Authority 5
HSA, see Health & Safety Authority 3–4

I

Ignition sources 83–84
Incidents 20–21 23 25 26 27
Injury statistics 1 14 15
Intoxicants 164
Infection Prevention & Control 72 115 117

L

Legislation 2–3 8 10 45 67 80 137 142
Lifestyle 150 157
Lone workers 44

M

Managing risk 155
Manual handling 7 34 36 44 68 74–77 148
Mechanical equipment 77–78
Mesothelioma 26
Microbiology 98

N

Needle stick injury 103
Night shift workers 45
NMBI, see Nursing and Midwifery Board of Ireland 5
Non-fatal accidents 24
Non-fatal injuries 24

O

Occupational deafness 26 34
Occupational diseases 26 71

INDEX

Occupational health risks 68–79
   Noise 68–69
   Fumes and dust 69–71
   Asthma 70–71
   Skin 71–73
Oxygen 7 59 83 86 88 103

P
Parasite 99 101 102 107
Pathogens 99
Personal Emergency Evacuation Plan (PEEP) 90–91
Personal injury 20 24
Pharmaceutical Society of Ireland (PSI) 5
Personal Protective Equipment (PPE) 19 39 122–129
   Aprons 127
   donning & removing 128
   facial protection 127
   footwear 128
   gloves 126
   users 124
   testing 125
   when to use 125
Prescribed medicines 165
Psychosocial hazards 50 53 56
   Violence at work 53–55
   Work-related stress 56–58

Q
Quaker Hill Nursing Home Fire 95–97

R
Radiation exposure 50
Radiological Protection Institute of Ireland (RPII) 5
Reactive monitoring 16
Reported incidents 14 21 74
Reporting and recording 23–27
   Accident investigations 26
   Keeping records 25
   Making a report 25
   Reporting an accident 25
Risk assessment 29–48
   Assessing risks 35
   Performing a risk assessment 33
   Risk, definition of 30
   Risk matrix 37
RPII, see Radiological Protection Institute of Ireland 5

S
Safety and healthy work practices 150 151 162
   Anti-bullying policy 40 151
   Grievance policy 151
Safety culture 151–152
Safety Data sheet 65–67
Safety management systems 26 146 151
Safety officers 7
Safety signs 92 132 133 172
   information signs 133 135
   mandatory signs 134
   prohibition signs 134
   warning signs 19 134
Safety Statement 9–12
   functions of 10
Safety, Health & Welfare at Work Act 2005 2
Slips, trips 2 14 18 21 40 51 154
Smoking 156 157
Spores 101 110

Spread of fire 84
Spread of micro-organisms 103–105
   direct contact 103
   indirect contact 103
Standard operating procedures 77
Standard precautions 115
   Airborne-based precautions 117
   Contact-based precautions 117
   Droplet-based precautions 118
   Transmission based precautions 116
Stress 35 53 55–57 69 162 165

T
Training 115 147–149 153 154
   AED 132
   Communication 136
   COVID-19 114
   Fire Safety 34 81 91 149
   First Aid 131
   HACCP and Food Safety 149
   Handover Communication 141
   Handwashing 73
   HIQA Compliance 149
   Manual Handling 39 76
   Mechanical Equipment 77
   PPE use 123–125
   Preventing Violence at work 54 55
   Sharps 39
Tuberculosis (TB) 100 109 113 117

V
Vibration 30 34 77
Violence 2 14 21 35 53 54 159
   Effects of 54
   Lone workers 44
   Work-related stress 56 57
Virus 98–100 137
   Blood-borne 111–113
Vulnerable groups 159

W
Work/life balance 157

Y
Younger workers 46–48

LIST OF LEGISLATION AND REGULATIONS

European Union (Personal Protective Equipment) Regulations 2018
Guide to the Safety, Health and Welfare at Work [General Application] Regulations 2007, Chapter 2 of Part 7: First Aid
Manual Handling of Loads Regulation
National Standards Authority of Ireland (NSAI) standards deal with emergency lighting (I.S. 3217) and fire alarm installation (I.S. 3218)
Protection of Young Persons (Employment) Act 1996
Safety Signs chapter of the General Application Regulations
Safety, Health and Welfare at Work (Biological Agents) Regulations 2013 (S.I. No. 572 of 2013)
Safety, Health and Welfare at Work (Carcinogens) Regulations 2019
Safety, Health and Welfare at Work (Chemical Agents) Regulations 2001
Safety, Health and Welfare at Work (General Application) Regulations 2016
Safety, Health and Welfare at Work (General Application) Regulations 2007
Safety, Health and Welfare at Work (General Application) Regulations 2007, Chapter 3 of Part 6: Night Work and Shift Work
Safety, Health and Welfare at Work (General Application) Regulations 2007, Chapter 4 of Part 2 (S.I. No. 299 of 2007)
Safety, Health and Welfare at Work (General Application) Regulations 2007 (Part 2, Chapter 3)
Safety, Health and Welfare at Work (Reporting of Accidents and Dangerous Occurrences) Regulations 2016 (S.I. No. 370 of 2016)
Safety, Health and Welfare at Work Act 2005
Schedule 3 of the Safety, Health and Welfare at Work (General Application) Regulations 2007
Section 8 of the Safety, Health and Welfare at Work 2005 Act
Section 9 of the Safety, Health and Welfare at Work Act 2005
Section 10 of the Safety, Health and Welfare at Work Act 2005

Section 11 of the Safety, Health and Welfare at Work Act 2005
Section 12 of the Safety, Health and Welfare at Work Act 2005
Section 13 (1) (b) of the Safety, Health and Welfare at Work Act 2005
Section 14 of the Safety, Health and Welfare at Work Act 2005
Section 19 of the Safety, Health and Welfare at Work Act 2005
Section 20 of the Safety, Health and Welfare at Work Act 2005
Section 25 of the Safety, Health and Welfare at Work Act 2005
Section 26 of the Safety, Health and Welfare at Work Act 2005
Workplace chapter of the Safety, Health and Welfare at Work (General Application) Regulations 2007 (the General Application Regulations)
Workplace chapter of the Safety, Health and Welfare at Work (General Application) Regulations 2007 (the General Application Regulations) details fire safety requirements as follows:
Regulation 11 – Doors and gates
Regulation 12 – Emergency routes and exits
Regulation 13 – Fire detection and firefighting
Regulation 25 – Employees with disabilities.